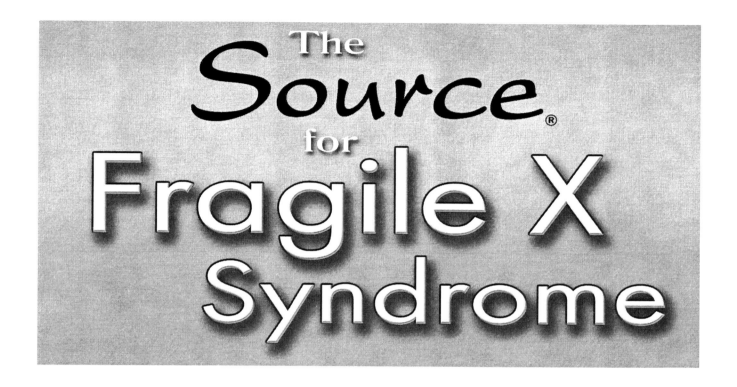

The Source for Fragile X Syndrome

Gail Harris-Schmidt
Dale Fast

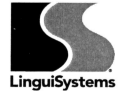

LinguiSystems

LinguiSystems, Inc.
3100 4th Avenue
East Moline, IL 61244

800-776-4332

FAX: 800-577-4555
E-mail: service@linguisystems.com
Web: linguisystems.com

| Interest Area: | Fragile X Syndrome |
| Ages: | Birth-21 |

Printed in the U.S.A.
ISBN 10: 0-7606-0520-3
ISBN 13: 978-0-7606-0520-2

About the Authors

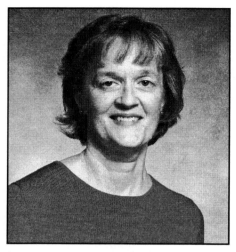

Gail Harris-Schmidt, Ph.D., CCC-SLP, is an Associate Professor and Department Chair of the Program in Communication Sciences and Disorders at Saint Xavier University in Chicago, where she has taught for the last 25 years. She received her Ph.D. in Learning Disabilities from Northwestern University and her M.A. in Speech-Language Pathology at Vanderbilt University. Previous to coming to Saint Xavier, she worked as a speech-language pathologist in the public schools and in a private school for children with learning disabilities. Gail received the Saint Xavier University Award in 2003, which honors a faculty member for service. She has presented numerous workshops on fragile X syndrome at national, state and local conferences, worked on the National Fragile X Foundation website, written a chapter for a special education textbook series, and served as a consultant to school districts regarding children with fragile X.

Gail and her husband Steve are the parents of two boys, one of whom has fragile X syndrome. They are all active in the Fragile X Resource Group of Greater Chicago and have worked on fundraisers, childcare at the last Foundation Conference, and family events. *The Source for Fragile X Syndrome* is Gail's first publication with LinguiSystems.

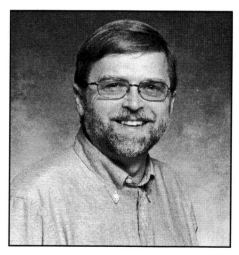

Dale Fast, Ph.D., is an Associate Professor of Biology at Saint Xavier University in Chicago where he teaches courses in general biology, AIDS, and genetics. In collaboration with Gail Harris-Schmidt, he has presented workshops on fragile X syndrome at many professional meetings and written a chapter for a special education text. In 2001, he received the Saint Xavier University Award for service. In 2002, he was awarded the National Fragile X Foundation Service Award for his work on the foundation's website.

After completing his undergraduate work at Tabor College, Dale taught high school in the Democratic Republic of Congo. Later, he received his Ph.D. from the University of Chicago where he studied yeast genetics, development, and biochemistry. He is an avid photographer, kayaker, and soccer fan, and also sings in his church choir. *The Source for Fragile X Syndrome* is Dale's first publication with LinguiSystems.

*T*able of *C*ontents

Acknowledgment

We are deeply grateful to the members of the Fragile X Resource Group of Greater Chicago and the speech-language pathologists who work with children having fragile X, who were interviewed for this book. We would also like to thank Ruth Fast, Claudia Harris, Joyce Jastrzab, Randolph Krohmer, Joanne Maczulski, Stephen Schmidt, and Maryann Shaunnessey for reading chapters of the manuscript and providing very helpful suggestions. Of course, they should not be held responsible for what we have written here. Our editor at LinguiSystems, Paul Johnson, has been creative, thorough, and patient throughout this project. We are grateful for his help in bringing this book to life. We have both been supported by numerous family members, colleagues, and friends, without whom this book could not have been written. Photographs of individuals used throughout the book were graciously shared by families in the Chicago area.

— Gail & Dale

Dedication

This book is dedicated to all of the families who have been affected by fragile X syndrome and to the special professionals who are working with them.

chapter 1 *Introduction*

An Unfamiliar Disease

Chicago's Red Moon Theater once gave a performance of Moby Dick. An actor walked out on the stage with two hand puppets. He said, "This is a story about a fight between a man and a whale. The whale won." Then the actor walked off the stage. Later, he and others returned to tell the story again in several versions with more detail. The story of fragile X syndrome can also be told in short and long versions. The short one sentence version is this: Fragile X syndrome is the leading cause of inherited neurodevelopmental disability. Many people respond to that statement by saying, "If it's that common, why haven't I ever heard about it?"

Fragile X syndrome is the leading cause of inherited neurodevelopmental disability.

Research

There are many reasons why people may not have heard of fragile X syndrome. For one thing, we have only recently learned about it. Martin and Bell (1943) first showed that this particular form of neurodevelopmental disability was X-linked and many years later, Lubs (1969) discovered that mentally retarded members of one family had an unusual constriction in their X chromosomes. A few dozen more articles were written about this X-linked gene in the 1970s.

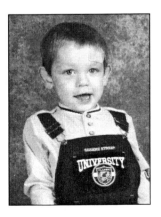

Despite those earlier mentions, most of the medical research on fragile X has occurred in the past 20 years. A search on PubMed at the National Library of Medicine shows that 620 research articles were published about fragile X syndrome in the 1980s. That number doubled in the 1990s, to 1281.

Fragile X has only appeared in educational research for a decade. A search of the ERIC database (Educational Resources Information Center) shows no entries about fragile X syndrome prior to 1994.

News Coverage

Another reason fragile X syndrome is not better known to the public is that it cannot easily be described in sound bytes. When you ask parents, caregivers, or researchers a question about fragile X, they often take a deep breath and try to decide if you really want to hear the complete story. Questions that are easy to answer about other diseases are often complicated when they relate to fragile X syndrome.

Questions that are easy to answer about other diseases are often complicated when they relate to fragile X syndrome.

Perhaps that is one of the reasons that fragile X syndrome has not been a major topic in the public press. A search of a collection of major newspapers shows that recently there were 55 articles on Asperger's syndrome, 263 on Down syndrome, 2,663 on breast cancer, and 15 articles on fragile X syndrome.

As you can see, if you don't know much about fragile X syndrome, it is simply because it is a relatively new area of study, and most people haven't had a lot of opportunities to learn about it.

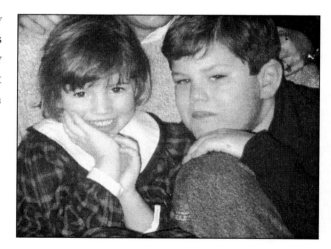

Diagnosis

Hodapp and colleagues (2003) note that the authors of a text on special education (Blackhurst & Berdine, 1993) argue that "classification systems based on etiology or clinical types have little value in education" (p. 425). This would suggest that there is little educational value in knowing whether the child is facing problems in the classroom because of fragile X syndrome, or because of some other reason.

Hodapp (2003) counters by arguing that it is possible to do etiology-based interventions. In subsequent chapters in this book, some of the interventions we suggest are generic interventions targeted at behaviors or difficulties that would be common to individuals with fragile X and many other syndromes. In other cases, however, research focused on individuals with fragile X syndrome has produced intervention models that specifically address the collage of strengths and weaknesses in individuals with the syndrome.

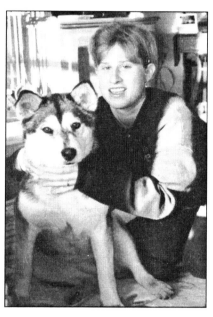

Diagnosis Missed or Delayed

Diagnosis of fragile X syndrome is often delayed, preventing the possibility of early intervention services and family planning. One survey of families who have a son with fragile X found that 24% had more than 10 visits to a health-care provider with concerns about their son's behavior and development before he was diagnosed with fragile X. Fifty percent of the families had another child before the first child with fragile X was diagnosed. Daughters with

Diagnosis of fragile X syndrome is often delayed, preventing the possibility of early intervention services and family planning.

fragile X are even less likely to be diagnosed at an early age (Bailey et al., 2002). Young children with fragile X may be misdiagnosed as having Prader-Willi syndrome, Sotos syndrome, Cohen syndrome, or isolated autism (Stoll, 2001).

Early Studies on X-Linked Inheritance

While most of the story of fragile X syndrome is only two decades old, some earlier work contributed to our understanding of this inherited disease.

X-Linked Genes

Morgan (1910) was the first to identify a gene located on the X chromosome, the gene for white eyes in the fruit fly, *Drosophila*. Later, it was shown that color blindness and hemophilia in humans are linked to the X chromosome.

X-Linked Mental Retardation

For many years, it has been known that there are more males with mental retardation than females (Goddard, 1914; Johnson, 1897). Males have only one X chromosome and thus receive only one copy of any X-linked gene that contributes to development and functioning of the brain. Females receive an X chromosome from each parent and thus are more likely to receive a working version of an X-linked gene that can cover up a defect in a non-working version of the gene. As a result, non-functioning genes located on the X chromosome are more likely to show up in males than in females.

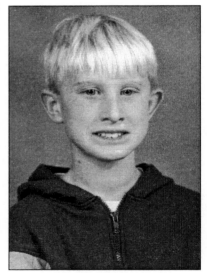

In the 1940s, researchers documented several examples of persons with severe mental retardation that exhibited a pattern of X-linked inheritance (Allan & Herndon, 1944; Allan, Herndon, & Dudley, 1944; Martin & Bell, 1943). Fragile X is but one of a collection of genes on the X chromosome that can cause mental retardation. These genes collectively are called *X-linked mental retardation* (XLMR) (Chiurazzi, Hamel, & Neri, 2001).

Variation in Fragile X Syndrome

Today we know that males and females with fragile X syndrome have a mutation on their X chromosome. It is a mutated form of the fragile X mental retardation gene, FMR1. These individuals have physical, behavioral, speech and language, sensory, and cognitive features that are a result of that mutation. We also know that among individuals with fragile X, there is a wide range of expression of those features.

This variation in features of the syndrome was not obvious in the research done prior to the identification in 1991 of the gene that causes fragile X (Verkerk et al., 1991). Early research on what we today identify as fragile X syndrome focused on families in which there were persons with severe retardation. Many of the first studies of fragile X syndrome looked at institutionalized males. As a result, the research overlooked many individuals who had more subtle impacts from fragile X.

Identification of Fragile X Syndrome

What we today call fragile X syndrome had a variety of early names. Titles of research articles referred to a marker X chromosome (Lubs, 1969), familial X-linked mental retardation with an X chromosome abnormality (Harvey, Judge, & Wiener, 1977), X-linked mental deficiency megalotestes syndrome (Ruvalcaba, Myhre, Roosen-Runge, & Beckwith, 1977), and Martin-Bell syndrome (Richards, Sylvester, & Brooker, 1981).

Early on, researchers wanted to know what proportion of males with severe retardation could be accounted for by X-linked genes, in particular the gene we now know causes fragile X. Since the method of screening for fragile X prior to the 1990's was difficult and expensive, people searched for ways to identify likely candidates. They looked for physical, behavioral, or chromosomal features that were also present in those individuals

> ### *Early Names for Fragile X*
>
> * familial X-linked mental retardation with an X chromosome abnormality
> * X-linked mental deficiency megalotestes syndrome
> * Martin-Bell syndrome

(Cantú et al., 1976; Giraud, Ayme, Mattei, & Mattei, 1976; Harvey et al., 1977; Lubs, 1969; Ruvalcaba et al., 1977; Turner et al., 1975). Eventually, a range of physical, cognitive, and behavioral features associated with fragile X was identified.

Overview

The previous sections contained the "short version" of the fragile X story. Following is the "medium-length" version.

Frequency

Individuals with fragile X syndrome have been found in every population that has been studied to date. Most studies find its prevalence in the general population to be about 1 in 4000 males and while the data are less clear, about 1 in 8000 females. It is estimated that 1 in 1000 males and 1 in 350 females has the premutation (discussed below) (Sherman, 2002).

Inheritance

The details of the inheritance of fragile X syndrome are described in **Chapter 9: Biological Basis** (page 117). Individuals with the common version of the fragile X mental retardation gene (FMR1) typically pass on the common version of the FMR1 gene to their offspring. These individuals do not have fragile X syndrome. In rare cases, though, they will have a child with a premutation in the FMR1 gene. The premutation has only limited impact on the individual. The future generations produced from this person with a premutation may experience continued change (mutation) in the FMR1 gene. Over several generations this can lead to a child with the full mutation. The final step moving from premutation to full mutation only occurs from mother to child; fathers do not give the full mutation to their children.

Individuals with the common version of the fragile X mental retardation gene (FMR1) typically pass on the common version of the FMR1 gene to their offspring.

A male with the full mutation will not produce the FMR protein. The absence of that protein will trigger significant cognitive, behavioral, and physical complications for him. A female with the full mutation will probably have fewer complications than would be seen in the male.

If this sounds complicated, that is because it is complicated. A working knowledge of this information will help you understand the factors that contribute to the complexity of this syndrome and its causes.

Physical Characteristics

The following physical characteristics are observed in many (but not all) males with the full mutation for fragile X syndrome. These characteristics are more likely to appear in males after puberty:

* long faces

* protruding ears

* large testicles

* problems with connective tissue that leads to flat feet, ear infections, and mitral valve prolapse in the heart

Males with the premutation may develop fragile X-associated tremor/ataxia syndrome (FXTAS).

Following puberty, some females with the full mutation will have long faces, protruding ears, and/or flat feet. They are less likely to exhibit these characteristics than males with the full mutation.

Females with the premutation may experience premature ovarian failure (early menopause). Physical characteristics are explored in greater depth in **Chapter 2: Physical Characteristics** (page 19).

The Rest of the Story

In the chapters summarized on the following pages, we will tell the long version of the story of fragile X syndrome. The major areas that may be affected by fragile X are explored for both boys and girls. Cognitive development, sensory issues, speech and language development, and behavior and emotional issues are examined in each of four chapters. Then the impact of these four areas on educational programming and placements and the teaching of academic areas are discussed. In the final chapters, a more in-depth biological explanation of fragile X syndrome is offered, and we conclude the book with future directions in research and intervention.

Chapter 3: Cognitive Development

Cognitive development is often affected for those with fragile X. Most boys who have the full mutation of fragile X have some level of cognitive impairment, with many scoring in the range of mental retardation. Girls with fragile X are usually less severely affected, but they may have mild mental retardation or specific learning disabilities.

Boys often show strengths in simultaneous processing, long term auditory memory, and visual memory. Weaknesses may be seen in sequential processing, abstract thinking, and arithmetic. Girls may have strengths in concrete verbal areas, with weaknesses in arithmetic and executive function tasks. Both boys and girls may have anxiety and attention issues — which affect IQ testing — so that their scores may not reflect their maximum potential.

Chapter 4: Sensory Issues

Sensory problems have been noted, even in very young children with fragile X syndrome. Parents may notice high arousal levels and hypersensitivity to sounds, light, touch, and textures when their child is an infant. Children may show tactile defensiveness, with strong negative reactions to being held or to various types of clothing. Some children with fragile X also have hyposensitivity, especially around the mouth, to the degree that they are very messy eaters. Sensory issues are important for occupational therapists and other members of the special education team to monitor, as classroom adaptations and calming techniques may need to be part of everyday planning.

Chapter 5: Speech and Language Development

Speech and language development is a significant area of weakness for most boys with fragile X. The lack of speech in these young boys is often the first indicator to parents that something is wrong developmentally with their child. For boys with fragile X, physical characteristics, cognitive levels, sensory issues, behaviors, and emotional development all affect speech and language.

Boys often have a history of recurrent ear infections and oral motor weaknesses that can affect both language comprehension and speech production. Language comprehension is usually in keeping with overall cognitive levels, although receptive vocabulary in areas of interest may be a strength. Expressively, boys may have a fast rate of speech, with cluttered, imprecise output. Pragmatics is a serious area of concern for most boys, as perseveration, poor eye contact, and impaired topic maintenance affect the ability to maintain a conversation.

For girls, speech and language may be relative areas of strength, but they may have difficulties in sequencing ideas, and because of their anxiety and shyness, with pragmatics. Language skills are generally in keeping with their cognitive levels and at a higher level than their mathematics and visual-spatial skills.

Chapter 6: Behavioral and Emotional Issues

A final area that affects overall development is that of behavior and emotional development. Behavioral outbursts, attention deficit/hyperactivity disorders (ADHD), and anxiety, along with autistic-like characteristics, are common to many boys with fragile X. Girls with fragile X often have significant issues with anxiety, sometimes accompanied by depression, and may have attention deficit/hyperactivity disorders of the predominantly inattentive type (ADHD-I). For these emotional and behavioral areas, an integrated plan of medical, behavioral, and therapeutic response needs to be in place.

Chapters 7 & 8: Educational Programming and Academic Intervention

In chapters 7 and 8, academic skill areas and settings are discussed in terms of effective programming and most appropriate placements for children with fragile X. Effective programs in early intervention, early childhood education, elementary, junior high, and high school settings are examined. Strategies for the academic areas of reading, written language, mathematics, science, social studies, and computer literacy are then presented.

Chapters 9 & 10: Biological Basis and Future Directions

We are beginning to understand how a mutation in a gene can result in significant neurodevelopmental problems. The final two chapters summarize what is currently known about the biological foundation of fragile X and look at some of the research that is pointing to future possibilities in addressing the challenges posed by fragile X syndrome.

chapter 2 *Physical Characteristics*

Why Study Physical Characteristics?

The most important impact of fragile X syndrome is the impact on the development and functioning of the brain. So why should one be interested in the impact of this syndrome on other parts of the body?

Screening

In the 1980s, it was very difficult to diagnose someone with fragile X. The chromosomal analysis required for a definitive diagnosis was expensive and not always reliable. As a result, many looked for physical or behavioral markers that could easily identify individuals who were likely to test positive for fragile X.

While diagnosis is easier to do today, we still look for simple ways to identify individuals who should be given the DNA test for fragile X. Professionals search for clues to help them differentiate among the myriad of possible causes of developmental disability.

. . . no one characteristic (other than the DNA test for fragile X) is a clear indicator that someone has fragile X syndrome.

The following pages describe a wide range of physical characteristics that appear more often in individuals with fragile X than in those who don't have fragile X. It should be noted, however, that there are many males with large protruding ears, flat feet, or hyperextensible finger joints (double jointedness) who do not have fragile X. There are also many females who experience early menopause who do not have fragile X. While there are characteristics that tend to show up in greater frequency in individuals with fragile X, no one characteristic (other than the DNA test for fragile X) is a clear indicator that someone has fragile X syndrome.

Early Warning

Fragile X may impact the development of the teeth, heart, feet, and other parts of the body. Once someone has been diagnosed with fragile X syndrome, caregivers and families can be alerted to possible areas of concern.

Possible Solutions

We are beginning to discover some of the biological underpinnings of cognitive and behavioral problems observed in individuals with fragile X syndrome. Understanding how the brain is processing things differently may lead to strategies for facilitating learning; understanding how connective tissue is different may help us address sensory issues.

Categories of Individuals with Fragile X

Before we can explore the range of physical characteristics seen in individuals with fragile X syndrome, we need to cluster individuals into groups. As we will discuss in detail in Chapter 9, people have many different versions of the gene that causes fragile X syndrome. For now, we will simply divide all people into 6 groups:

* ✳ males who have the full mutation for fragile X
* ✳ females who have the full mutation for fragile X
* ✳ males who have a premutation for fragile X
* ✳ females who have a premutation for fragile X
* ✳ males who don't have fragile X
* ✳ females who don't have fragile X

Males With the Full Mutation

The individuals most significantly impacted by fragile X are the males with the full mutation. As we will discuss later, these individuals will experience significant behavioral and cognitive effects from fragile X. Similarly, they are the ones most likely to display physical effects from the mutation.

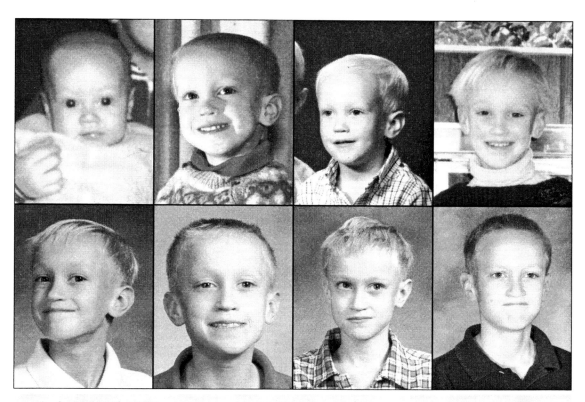

growth of a boy with fragile X syndrome

✳ Head

Identifying infants and toddlers who should be tested for fragile X syndrome based on facial features is difficult (Bailey, Roberts, Mirrett, & Hatton, 2001). Nevertheless, there are some features that may be evident prior to puberty. Young boys with the full mutation often have broad palpebral fissures (from one corner of the eyelid to the other) and as a result, narrow inner canthal distances (from the corner of one eyelid to the corner of the other eyelid) (Butler, Allen, Singh, Carpenter, & Hall, 1988). Some will have puffy eyelids resulting in a narrowing of the opening of the eye from top to bottom (Hockey & Crowhurst, 1988). Strabismus, difficulty directing the eyes to the same object, is another observed feature (Storm, PeBenito, & Ferretti, 1987).

The circumference of the head in boys is somewhat larger than usual (Partington, 1984). Some may have large and/or protruding ears, a long face and a high, arched palate (Simko, Hornstein, Soukup, & Bagamery, 1989). This latter characteristic may have speech-related implications. There may also be an acceleration in dental maturity in children (Kotilainen & Pirinen, 1999). The physical features that most people associate with fragile X syndrome in adult males are prominent ears and a long face. Postpubertal males with fragile X often (but not always) have long ears, wide ears, and long head (Butler, Pratesi, Watson, Breg, & Singh, 1993; Lisik, Szymanska-Parkieta, & Galecka, 2000; Loesch & Sampson, 1993). The crown teeth may show size asymmetry (Peretz et al., 1988).

* Brain
The impact of fragile X on the brain will be addressed in several chapters in this book. Fragile X affects behavior, cognition, and physiological responses. In some cases, there is a documented biological underpinning that causes these impacts. For example, there is research on the physiological responses to sounds. In control males, repetitions of identical tones results in a decrease in the brain's response to the stimulus. In boys with fragile X, the initial response was larger and repetitions did not lead to diminished responses (Castrén, Pääkkönen, Tarkka, Ryynänen, & Partanen, 2003).

Epilepsy is present in 20-25% of males with the full mutation, but it often disappears before the age of 20 (Sabaratnam, Vroegop, & Gangadharan, 2001). EEGs of both those with epilepsy and those without, may show a variety of abnormalities (Berry-Kravis, 2002). Those that demonstrate abnormal EEGs are more likely to have seizures at a later time (Berry-Kravis, 2002). This may allow us to identify individuals at high risk for seizures. Chapter 9 addresses some of the impacts of fragile X on the structural development of neurons.

* Physiological Arousal
Studies on heart rate variability suggest that boys with fragile X may have modified physiological responses that provide a biological basis for some of the behavior regulation problems they experience. They have higher levels of heart activity during passive phases, and the sympathetic and parasympathetic systems do not appear to be well coordinated (Roberts, Boccia, Bailey, Hatton, & Skinner, 2001).

✳ Connective Tissue

There are a number of characteristics in males with the full mutation that appear to be related to connective tissue abnormalities (Opitz, Westphal, & Daniel, 1984). Some have primary cutis verticis gyrata (a furrowing of the scalp) (Schepis et al., 1990), recurrent otitis media (ear infections) (Hagerman, Altshul-Stark, & McBogg, 1987), flat feet (Davids, Hagerman, & Eilert, 1990), and hyperextensibility of finger joints (double-jointedness) (Hagerman, Van Housen, Smith, & McGavran, 1984).

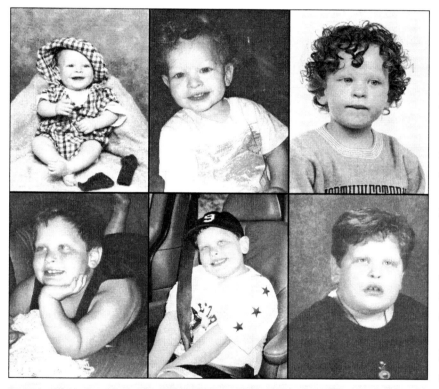

facial and body changes in a boy with fragile X syndrome

Some individuals with fragile X have mitral valve prolapse, which results in a click or murmur in the heart. Others have dilation of the aorta that can lead to the weakening of that blood vessel (Hagerman & Synhorst, 1984). These cardiovascular abnormalities are not seen as often in children but appear later in development (Crabbe, Bensky, Hornstein, & Schwartz, 1993).

The soft skin that is frequently observed in these individuals may be the result of collagen or elastin abnormalities (Waldstein et al., 1987). This may be one of the biological underpinnings that result in significant sensory issues for these individuals.

✳ Body

A subgroup of males with fragile X will have extreme obesity, a round face, and small, broad hands and feet that may be misdiagnosed as Prader-Willi syndrome. This increase in body dimensions occurs between the ages of 5 and 10 (de Vries et al., 1993). Some other children with fragile X exhibit general overgrowth typical of the classical Sotos syndrome (de Vries et al., 1995).

Adult males often have small stature and disproportionately shorter limbs with enlarged chest and waist (Loesch, Lafranchi, & Scott, 1988). In the development of bones in the hands, ossification is delayed and abnormal (Kjaer, Hjalgrim, & Russell, 2001). Some individuals have scoliosis (Davids et al., 1990).

* Macroorchidism
Adult males with fragile X typically have testicles with 2-3 times the volume of that seen in males without fragile X (Butler, Brunschwig, Miller, & Hagerman, 1992). Enlargement of the testicles (macroorchidism) is also common among males who are mentally retarded who do not have fragile X (Cossée et al., 1997), so by itself, it is not diagnostic for fragile X. Mice in which the FMR1 gene has been inactivated, also produce enlarged testes (Slegtenhorst-Eegdeman et al., 1998).

Most human males with the full mutation do not reproduce. However, some do have children, so the macroorchidsm does not result in sterility. The sons will, of course, receive a Y chromosome from the father, and curiously, the daughters receive an X chromosome with a reduced number of repeats, not the full mutation (Laird, 1991).

Macroorchidism is less frequent among pre-pubertal boys and if it does develop, it often does not appear before the age of 8 (Lachiewicz & Dawson, 1994).

* Mortality
One report suggested that there might be an increased rate of sudden infant death in children of females with the full mutation (Fryns, Moerman, Gilis, d'Espallier, & Van den Berghe, 1988). Authors of another study concluded that life expectancy among adults with the full mutation is similar to that in the general population (Partington, Robinson, Laing, & Turner, 1992). In fact, there is evidence that those with the full mutation have decreased rates of cancer (Schultz-Pedersen, Hasle, Olsen, & Friedrich, 2001).

Females With the Full Mutation

Perhaps the most notable observation about adult females with the full mutation is the diminished presence of features seen in males with the full mutation. Many of the features that do appear are less prominent than in males. If the features appear in females, they are more likely in adults than in children.

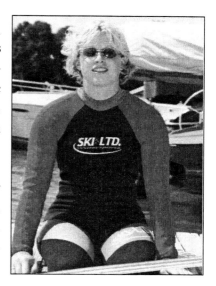

For example, some females with the full mutation do show an increase in ear prominence (Hull & Hagerman, 1993); however, they are less likely than males to have long and protruding ears. As in males, this feature is more common in adults than in children (Loesch & Hay, 1988).

Females with the full mutation are more likely than controls to have a high arched palate, double-jointed thumbs, and flat feet (Riddle, Cheema, & Sobesky, 1998). Several cases of precocious puberty have been found (Kowalczyk et al., 1996). Seizures are less frequent than in males with the full mutation (Berry-Kravis, 2002)

Males with the Pre-Mutation

Until recently, it was thought that the pre-mutation had no impact on males directly. Its only impact appeared to be that these individuals could have grandchildren with the full mutation. In recent years, it has become clear that the pre-mutation triggers fragile X-associated tremor/ataxia syndrome (FXTAS) in some males. This syndrome has no impact during childhood. It appears in some men who are over 50 years of age as a progressive neurological disorder. They experience cerebellar ataxia (irregularity of voluntary muscular movement) and/or intention (when voluntary motion is attempted) tremor. There may be other impacts on cognition and muscular function (Jacquemont et al., 2003). Postmortem studies on brains of men with tremor/ataxia show a variety of histological abnormalities (Greco et al., 2002).

It is noteworthy that this condition does not appear in females with the pre-mutation nor in males or females with the full mutation. Researchers have documented that males with the pre-mutation overproduce the messenger RNA for the fragile X protein (Tassone, Hagerman, Taylor et al., 2000). It may be that these elevated messenger RNAs have a toxic effect leading to the tremor/ataxia (Hagerman et al., 2001).

Females with the Pre-Mutation

Females with the pre-mutation continue to produce the FMR protein, albeit at lowered levels. They do produce elevated levels of the messenger RNA for the FMR protein, indicating that the messenger RNA is not working efficiently (Tassone, Hagerman, Chamberlain, & Hagerman, 2000). Since they do produce the FMR protein, one might expect to find no impact from the expanded number of repeats. Nevertheless, some features appear.

Females with the pre-mutation for fragile X exhibit few physical manifestations of the syndrome. They are more likely to have prominent ears than controls (Hull & Hagerman, 1993) and more likely to have a prominent jaw (Riddle, Cheema, Sobesky et al., 1998).

The primary physical impact on females with the pre-mutation is premature ovarian failure (POF), or early menopause. In one study, 16% of the females with the pre-mutation experienced menopause prior to the age of 40. Curiously this does not occur in females with the full mutation (Allingham-Hawkins et al., 1999).

Females with the premutation showed no significant difference in occurrence of diseases commonly associated with menopause, such as cardiovascular diseases and osteoporosis. Some of those with premature ovarian failure did have lower bone mineral density (Hundscheid, Smits, Thomas, Kiemeney, & Braat, 2003).

Some researchers have found an increase in twinning, particularly among those with POF (Vianna-Morgante, 1999), while others do not see a similar pattern (Murray, Ennis, MacSwiney, Webb, & Morton, 2000).

Summary

As you have seen in this chapter, the physical impacts of fragile X syndrome on a person are limited. If the FMR1 gene did not impact the cognitive, behavioral, and sensory characteristics of a person, it would not generate significant interest. There would not be such a massive focus on research about fragile X if it simply caused big ears, long faces, and velvety skin.

Nevertheless, as you will see in the following chapters, some of the physical characteristics of fragile X, such as connective tissue problems, physiological responses, and high arched palate, may help us understand the biological basis of sensory, behavioral, and speech challenges faced by persons with fragile X syndrome.

chapter 3 Cognitive Development

Characteristics

Fragile X syndrome plays a major role in the cognitive development of those with the full genetic mutation. Most research articles on fragile X begin with sentences such as, "Fragile X syndrome is considered to be the most common inherited cause of mental retardation" or "Fragile X syndrome is the leading inherited cause of developmental disabilities." As discussed in Chapter 1, fragile X syndrome has a less dramatic effect on females than it does on males; however, the range of cognitive development is broad for both males and females. Estimates of the numbers of those diagnosed with fragile X who fall into various levels of cognitive functioning are inconsistent. The lack of consistency results from many factors, such as the specific populations studied, the diagnostic instruments used, and the reality that the fragile X diagnosis has become more widely recognized in recent years (Bennetto and Pennington, 2002).

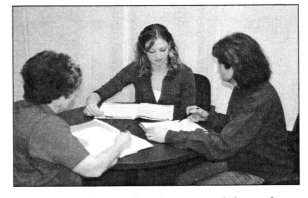

The samples chosen for study range from those in institutionalized settings to those in inclusive settings, from those in early childhood to senior citizens, from those diagnosed with autism to those who are not, from those who have spoken language to those who do not, and from those with the full genetic mutation to those with the premutation. A wide array of intelligence tests, including the Wechsler scales (Wechsler, 1974, 1981), the *Stanford-Binet* (Thorndike, Hagen, and Sattler, 1985) and the *Kaufman-ABC* (Kaufman and Kaufman, 1983), with many types of demands, have been used in the studies, and a number of areas, including anxiety, sensory, and attention deficit disorders, affect the scores on IQ tests of persons who have fragile X.

General Abilities in Boys

In 1992, Santos estimated that 30 percent of males with fragile X functioned in the severe/profound range of mental retardation, with 60 percent in the mild/moderate range, and 10 percent in the borderline/low normal range. She stated that as more mildly involved boys are identified as having fragile X syndrome, the numbers were likely to change. In 1995, Freund, Peebles, Aylward, and Reiss stated that 44 percent of boys functioned in the borderline to normal range on the *Stanford-Binet Scales of Intelligence* (Thorndike, Hagen, and Sattler, 1985). Bennetto and Pennington (2002) believe that most adult males with fragile X score in the moderate to severe range of mental retardation, but that there may be a continuum of involvement in fragile X syndrome depending upon the degree of FMR1 protein that is produced.

While many people with fragile X seem to have autistic-like characteristics, most do not meet all of the diagnostic criteria . . . for autism.

Several studies have been specifically designed to analyze the relationship of fragile X to autism and that connection to cognitive development. While many people with fragile X seem to have autistic-like characteristics, most do not meet all of the diagnostic criteria of the Diagnostic Statistical Manual-IV (American Psychiatric Association, 1994) for autism. But, a significant minority of boys with fragile X, with estimates from 10 to 33 percent, meet the diagnostic criteria for autism (Feinstein and Reiss, 1998; Rogers, Wehner, and Hagerman, 2001). Among children with fragile X, this group of children seems to have the most serious difficulties in the area of language and cognition, with scores at the lower end of the cognitive range (Bailey, Hatton, Skinner, and Mesibov, 2001).

Specific Abilities in Boys

Although boys with fragile X syndrome may show a wide range of abilities, there are similarities in their patterns on many cognitive measures. Much of the research literature speaks of strengths in simultaneous processing, long term memory, visual memory, and verbal imitation, with weaknesses in sequential processing, abstract thinking and reasoning, short term memory, verbal response and recall, problem solving, selective attention, and fine motor skills (Braden, 2000b; Kemper, Hagerman, and Altshul-Stark, 1988; Saunders, 2001; Schoenbrodt and Smith, 1995; Spiridigliozzi, Lachiewicz, MacMurdo, Vizoso, O'Donnell, Conkie-Russell, and Burgess, 1994).

Simultaneous processing involves the integration of stimuli to form a whole image, while sequential processing involves putting a series of steps together to form a whole. Children with simultaneous processing strengths can learn and retain whole images, but if they lack sequential processing abilities, they often have difficulty putting parts in order. They may have difficulty recognizing previously learned information if a part of that whole is omitted (Braden, 2000b; Saunders, 2001). Sequential processing is needed to follow directions in order, to sound out a word, to repeat a series of numbers, or to put ideas or pictures in order to tell a story. Weaknesses in sequential processing may cause boys with fragile X to have difficulty when taught by a "part to whole" method, such as the use of phonics to teach reading or the explanation of steps to complete a task without first showing the finished product.

Strengths in Boys with Fragile X

* simultaneous processing
* long-term memory
* visual memory
* verbal imitation

Weaknesses in Boys with Fragile X

* sequential processing
* abstract thinking and reasoning
* short-term memory
* verbal response and recall
* problem solving
* selective attention
* fine motor skills

General Abilities in Girls

Girls who inherit the fragile X gene from their fathers usually have the premutation instead of the full mutation of the gene and are rarely mentally impaired. Those who inherit the gene from their mothers may have the full mutation, resulting in learning disabilities or mild mental retardation, but they may have only the premutation with no cognitive impairments. It is estimated that anywhere from 25 to 50 percent of females with the full mutation have borderline or below normal IQ scores (Schoenbrodt and Smith, 1995; DeVries, Wiegers, Smits, Mohkamsing, Duivenvoorden, Fryns, Curfs, Halley, Oostra, van den Ouweland, and Niermeijer, 1996). In the DeVries et al. study, 57 percent of the women with the full mutation had IQs 30 points or more below those of their unaffected sisters. Many girls are diagnosed with nonverbal learning disabilities, which particularly affect mathematics and pragmatics skills, such as social perception.

It is estimated that anywhere from 25 to 50 percent of females with the full mutation have borderline or below normal IQ scores.

Research studies have consistently shown that in terms of cognitive development, there are no differences between premutation carriers of the fragile X syndrome and those unaffected by fragile X (Brainard, Schreiner, and Hagerman, 1991; Myers, Mazzocco, Maddalena, and Reiss, 2001). These findings may have implications for educators who work with the mothers of children with fragile X, as the mothers may or may not have cognitive difficulties themselves.

Specific Abilities in Girls

Girls who have the full mutation of the fragile X gene have some unique patterns in their performance on intelligence tests. On the Wechsler scales, Brainard, Schreiner, and Hagerman (1991) found strengths in the areas of vocabulary, comprehension, and digit symbol, with weaknesses in arithmetic. Other researchers cite difficulties in block design, a more abstract visual spatial task. These researchers also note difficulties in various nonverbal areas of learning, such as problem solving involving the executive function (Mazzocco, Hagerman, and Pennington, 1992; Sobesky, Pennington, Porter, Hull, and Hagerman, 1994). Bennetto, Pennington, Porter, Taylor, and Hagerman (2001) believe that executive function disorders, rather than visual spatial deficits, result from the full mutation of the fragile X gene in girls and women.

Diagnosis of Intelligence

Many researchers suggest using the *Kaufman Assessment Battery for Children* (K-ABC) (Kaufman and Kaufman, 1983) as the intelligence quotient measure for children with fragile X, as it divides tasks and scales into simultaneous and sequential processing areas and also provides both aptitude and achievement measures. The distinction between simultaneous and sequential processing is particularly important in testing boys, as Kemper, Hagerman, and Altshul-Stark (1988) found boys with fragile X to score an average of ten points higher on the simultaneous as opposed to the sequential portion of the test. Boys showed strengths in long-term memory and perceptual closure (Gestalt Closure), while scoring most poorly on visual-motor memory (Hand Movements), visual-spatial memory (Spatial Memory) and arithmetic. Kemper et al. (1988) also found that boys with fragile X scored better on the achievement portion of the test than they did on the aptitude portion, as their long-term memory for learned information (crystallized knowledge) served them well.

The distinction between simultaneous and sequential processing is particularly important in testing boys.

Other IQ measures have been used to study children with fragile X, with similar results. For example, when the *Stanford-Binet Scales of Intelligence* (Thorndike, Hagen, and Sattler, 1985) were used to assess boys with fragile X, strengths were found in verbal labeling and comprehension, with weaknesses in visual-motor coordination, spatial memory, and arithmetic (Freund and Reiss, 1991). Maes, Fryns, Van Wallenghem, and Van den Berghe (1994) used the *McCarthy Scales* (McCarthy, 1972) and found strengths in crystallized knowledge (word meanings) and with meaningful information, with weaknesses in less meaningful or abstract items (e.g., random digit strings).

For boys with mental retardation, some researchers (Smith, 1983) report a higher Verbal than Performance IQ on the Wechsler (1974, 1981) measures, while others (Fisch, 1993) find that the Verbal-Performance gap is not always present. Boys' weaknesses are usually found in digit span, arithmetic, and block design (Fisch, 1993), thinking and problem-solving skills, formulation of verbal responses on demand, motor planning tasks, (Spiridigliozzi, Lachiewicz, MacMurdo, Vizoso, O'Donnell, Conkie-Russell, and Burgess, 1994), sequential processing, arithmetic, and abstract reasoning (Schoenbrodt and Smith, 1995).

There is not extensive literature on the intelligence profiles of higher functioning boys with fragile X, particularly those with specific learning disabilities. There is likely an underdiagnosis of fragile X syndrome in the population of boys with fragile X. Boys with borderline or low normal IQs may have similar characteristics to those who score in the levels of mental retardation, with specific problems in higher level thinking skills, language, mathematics, and visual motor coordination.

[Girls'] specific learning disabilities often appear in the areas of mathematics and pragmatics, or social skills.

Girls with fragile X syndrome, as a group, have higher scores on IQ measures than do boys with fragile X. Girls often show a Verbal-Performance gap on measures such as the Wechsler scales, with particularly low scores in block design, arithmetic, and digit span. They often show strengths in rote verbal skills. Thus, girls may be good readers, with overall adequate skills in literal comprehension. Their specific learning disabilities often appear in the areas of mathematics and pragmatics, or social skills.

Girls may also be penalized on timed aspects of IQ tests, as they seem to trade speed for accuracy (Tamm, Menon, Johnston, Hessl, and Reiss, 2002).

Processing Levels

Processing problems affect the areas of cognition and achievement in many ways and also need to be assessed. Using Johnson and Myklebust's (1967) hierarchy of information processing, as adapted by Wren (1983), the areas where breakdowns may occur are defined. These authors do not see the hierarchy as strictly bottom up, but rather emphasize that any level of the hierarchy may affect other levels, either up or down the processing hierarchy. For instance, metacognitive strategies may be used to help memory, or attention strategies may be taught to help perception. Wilding, Cornish, and Muner's (2002) definitions of executive functioning are also appropriate to examine in relation to children who have fragile X syndrome. There is far less available research on girls with fragile X than there is on boys, but some areas of processing are mentioned in the literature (Bennetto, Pennington, Porter, Taylor, and Hagerman, 2001).

Hierarchy of Experience

Sensation	Receipt of data from eyes, ears, and touch
Attention	Focus upon the incoming sensations, and filtering of incoming data
Perception:	Discrimination of stimulus
Memory:	Short-term and long-term storage
Symbolization:	Attachment of meaning to perceptions
Conceptualization:	Classification or categorization of information
Metacognition:	Conscious awareness and manipulation of strategies and rules
Executive functioning:	Problem-solving and ability to flexibly modify strategies

based on Johnson and Myklebust, 1967; Wilding, Cornish, and Muner, 2002; Wren, 1983

✳ Attention

Most boys with fragile X syndrome are diagnosed with attention deficit disorder and are found to have significant problems in distractibility, impulsivity and hyperactivity. Their selective attention for relevant information may be very poor. Underlying attention problems may affect not only scores on IQ measures, but also performance on many learning tasks. Girls may have attention deficit disorders, but primarily of the inattentive type. Since girls do not as often exhibit hyperactivity and impulsivity, their attention problems may not be as noticeable in the classroom, or they may be thought to be having petit mal seizures.

* Perception

Perceptual problems may also affect learning. With their histories of recurrent ear infections, boys with fragile X may have perceptual (auditory discrimination) difficulties and may be unable to hear the differences among sounds. This may result in difficulties in comprehending and following directions, following conversations, and matching sounds to letters for reading.

* Memory

Memory is an interesting area of processing for both boys and girls with fragile X. While they may have difficulty with short-term memory, once information has been stored in long-term memory, it can be retrieved well. Long-term memory for many kinds of information is often seen as a strength by both parents and educators. The perseverative nature of the speech of boys with fragile X reflects this type of long-term memory store. Boys can often recall and repeat lines from videos and TV shows and recall exact scripts from various sources. This strength in long term-memory may be used in academic settings to increase children's knowledge bases.

* Symbolization

Symbolic processing may be an area of weakness for children with fragile X syndrome. While concrete facts may be learned with relative ease, more abstract concepts are difficult for them to grasp. In keeping with their cognitive levels, both boys and girls may find higher level thinking areas to be problematic. Children with fragile X are often able to memorize facts in areas such as science and social studies, but because they have not attached meaning to the facts that they are storing in memory, they may not be able to respond when questions are reworded or presented in a different manner.

* Conceptualization

  At the higher levels of processing, the area of conceptualization, or generalization, may be particularly difficult. Many children in special education settings have difficulty generalizing that which they have learned to new settings. This involves abstract processing, finding connections, and problem solving, all of which may be areas of weakness for children with fragile X.

* Metacognition

  Metacognitive processing has to do with a person's ability to think about his or her own thinking, to consider options for problem solving, to organize strategies, and to analyze results. This high level of processing may be very difficult for those with cognitive impairments, but some levels of self-reflection may be possible for higher functioning children who are specifically taught self-reflection strategies.

* Executive Functioning

  In a similar self-monitoring way, executive functioning, the ability to direct and switch attention, inhibit repetitive behavior, and inhibit inappropriate responses, is often cited as an area of difficulty for both boys and girls with fragile X (Wilding, Cornish, and Munir, 2002). Bennetto et al. (2002) found a striking deficiency in executive functioning in women with fragile X, independent of overall IQ level. They state that this weakness particularly affects fluid intelligence, the ability to problem solve in the face of novel information or situations.

Measuring IQ Over Time

While normally developing individuals without fragile X syndrome continue to develop their reasoning skills throughout their adolescent years, a decline in IQ is reported for some adolescents with fragile X. Research regarding declining IQs involves many problems, particularly with the methodologies employed. In a methodological critique of the research on IQ decline, Hay (1994) cites a number of problems in the studies. Data have been combined inappropriately using different IQ tests and age range normative samples, task demands in the tests, and models of intelligence. The tests that are best at discriminating around the population average are limited in their application to persons of low ability. In part,

The tests that are best at discriminating around the population average are limited in their application to persons of low ability.

this stems from insufficient sampling of persons at the extremes when norming IQ tests. In addition, specific behavioral (attentional, sensory) and cognitive deficits in fragile X individuals may confound the task demands of particular IQ tests at particular ages. Hay also states that most of the studies are cross-sectional rather than longitudinal, making comparisons difficult.

In a retrospective study of longitudinal changes in IQ scores of both boys and girls with fragile X syndrome, 28 percent of males and 36 percent of females were found to have significant declines (Wright-Talamante, Cheema, Riddle, Luckey, Taylor, and Hagerman, 1996). Ten of 35 males (28%) with the greatest decline were the males with mosaicism. These researchers believe that the IQ decline they found was due to difficulties in abstract reasoning, as the task demands of IQ tests shift upwards, and possibly to endocrine factors related to the onset of puberty. In fact, it may be that there are two types of fragile X mutations, one of which is static, in which no such declines would be seen, and the other, dynamic (Fisch, Shapiro, Simensen, Schwartz, Fryns, Borghgraef, Curfs, Howard-Peebles, Arinami, and Mavrou, 1992).

It is important for educators and parents to understand that the decline in IQ is more of a deceleration in cognitive development, rather than any type of degeneration of the central nervous system.

It is important for educators and parents to understand that the decline in IQ is more of a deceleration in cognitive development, rather than any type of degeneration of the central nervous system. Adolescents do not lose the skills and knowledge that they had acquired; rather, their rate of learning slows, and the abstract demands of more advanced IQ tests and upper level academics cannot be met.

Issues in Assessment

A number of issues need to be kept in mind when assessing the intelligence of children with fragile X. As explored in other chapters, many, if not most, children with fragile X face issues regarding anxiety, sensory overload, and attention. Therefore, children with fragile X syndrome may not show their maximum ability on formal IQ tests. Changes in routine are very difficult for them. The effect of an unfamiliar psychologist in an unfamiliar setting may result in negative outcomes on the measures. Taking a child away from the familiar routine of the classroom in order to test that child may provoke anxiety and less than optimal performance.

Evaluators need to provide calming activities before testing and use pictures or schedules to inform the children as to how many tasks there will be.

Evaluators need to provide calming activities before testing and use pictures or schedules to inform the children as to how many tasks there will be. Structured, calm testing situations with numerous breaks and rewards may be necessary. Cognition in children with fragile X is an area that must be assessed with the areas of sensory, language, and behavioral/emotional issues in mind. Adaptations of formal tests, informal testing, probes, and indirect questioning may provide more helpful results and accurate information. Authentic assessment measures (based upon relevant curriculum) and portfolios may do a better job of assessing the levels at which many individuals with fragile X are functioning. While it may be necessary to attain IQ levels for some initial placements, these may not be the numbers that provide the most helpful information for planning intervention.

Intervention

While no intervention can cure a cognitive disorder for a child or adolescent with fragile X syndrome, intervention can make a profound difference in the aptitude and achievements of children with fragile X. Early intervention in zero to three programs and early childhood special education programming, when cognitive growth may progress most rapidly, are vital for helping persons with fragile X syndrome to achieve their maximum potential.

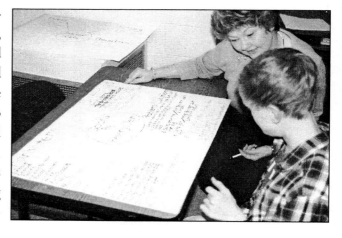

In a survey conducted by researchers at the University of North Carolina, it was found that someone, usually the mother, became concerned about her child's development at around eight to ten months of age. It was not until about 22 months that the child was diagnosed as developmentally delayed and enrolled in an early intervention program. It was still another year before many of those children were diagnosed as having fragile X syndrome (average 35 months) (www.fpg.unc.edu/~FX/Pages/findings). Thus, intervention, coupled with the knowledge provided by a diagnosis of etiology, was not available until the child was nearly three years old.

Early interventionists who were surveyed in these studies recommended programming that included these elements:

* specific behavioral plans

* a focus on attention

* work with sensory dysfunction and autistic-like characteristics

* speech-language intervention

* close collaboration with parents.

One of the major recommendations that emerged from the early intervention study was the need for professionals to work closely with parents to develop and implement behavioral plans and to work with the teaching of skills and concepts (www.fpg.unc.edu/~FX/Pages/findings). Early interventionists in the North Carolina studies appeared to be more concerned about behavioral issues in young children than about cognitive delays.

Intervention in the area of cognition needs to build on children's cognitive strengths, with mindfulness of the other areas of importance to their learning style, including sensory, speech-language, and behavioral/emotional issues. It is especially important to build a team with expertise in various areas to develop the Individual Family Service Plan (IFSP) and later, the Individual Educational Plan (IEP). Occupational therapists, speech-language pathologists, developmental specialists, physical therapists, special educators, psychologists, social workers, and parents all need to be involved in the team.

Intervention in the area of cognition needs to build on children's cognitive strengths, with mindfulness of the other areas of importance to their learning style . . .

Researchers at Stanford University have emphasized the importance of environmental as well as genetic influences on the cognitive outcomes of children with fragile X, and they recommend training parents and providers in skills essential for the children's maximum development. Dyer-Friedman, Glaser, Hessl, Johnston, Huffman, Taylor, Wisbeck, and Reiss (2002) found that both biological (amount of protein produced) and environmental factors predicted outcomes of children with the full mutation of the fragile X gene. They found that the cognitive outcome for girls was strongly predicted by the mean IQ of their parents, with a smaller amount of the variance predicted by the quality of their environment. For boys, mean parental IQ was associated with their Performance IQ, and the quality of their home environments accounted for more of the variance in their cognitive outcomes than it did for the girls.

In order to maximize the strength in modeling that many children with fragile X have, programming with regular education peers can be very beneficial. In early intervention settings and early childhood classes, it is common for all of the children to have special needs; however, if there are children in the classes who have spoken language and good play and social skills, they can be excellent models for the children with fragile X. In elementary school and beyond, it may be appropriate to spend some part of the day with regular education peers in inclusionary settings in order to maximize the opportunities for modeling.

Other principles for optimizing cognitive development will be expanded upon in the chapters on speech and language, behavior, academic, and sensory issues. These include:

* awareness of sensory issues
* use of calming techniques
* importance of schedules, routines
* need for visual cueing: pictures, logos, words
* focus on concrete, experiential learning
* emphasis on functional language
* teaching through high interest areas
* emphasis on simultaneous processing tasks before sequential

Conclusions

Cognitive development is clearly one of the areas most affected by fragile X syndrome. Most boys with the full genetic mutation are diagnosed with mental retardation, but the range of functioning is broad, and many possess learning strengths as well as weaknesses. Overall, girls with the full mutation have higher IQ levels than do boys, but they, too, present levels of cognitive ability across a wide range. In this chapter, the area of cognition, and its assessment and intervention, was explored in relation to many of the common characteristics of fragile X. Cognitive development is clearly an area where knowledge of etiology may affect the ways we assess and treat children with fragile X syndrome.

chapter 4

Sensory Issues

Characteristics of Sensory Development

Sensory issues may affect every other area of development for both boys and girls with fragile X syndrome. Cognition, speech and language, and behavior cannot be assessed or treated without attention to sensory issues. Hypersensitivity, with strong reactions to lights, noise, and touch, may be found in many children with fragile X. Avoidance of sensory experiences may then be associated with lower levels of school participation, play, and self-care (Baranek, Chin, Hess, Yankee, Hatton, and Hooper, 2002). There is also evidence of hyposensitivity, as seen in self-stimulation and poor eating and drinking skills.

Ayers' (1979) theory of sensory integration is often cited as an explanation for what children with fragile X are feeling. She believes that those with poor sensory integration do not consistently process and integrate the sensory input that they are receiving. Instead of their brains rapidly sorting, ordering, and translating sensory inputs into actions and reactions, children with fragile X must process a confused set of inputs, which often results in poor motor planning, confused language processing, and an inability to filter the relevant from the irrelevant. As Saunders (2001) states, Ayers' theory is controversial because her descriptions of brain activity are unproven, but the problems described as part of sensory integration disorders and the need for intervention regarding sorting out and dealing with multiple, overwhelming inputs fit the profile of many children with fragile X.

Hyperarousal

Sensory problems have been noticed even in very young children with fragile X. Hyperarousal may be the result of a defect in the autonomic nervous system, which results in a number of issues (Belser and Sudhalter, 1995, 2001). In infancy, hyperarousal problems may affect both sleep and touch.

Parents often report problems with their children's sleep cycles, particularly with children awakening in the night or waking up extremely early. Difficulties with falling or staying asleep seem to persist long past the time that other children are sleeping through the night. It is possible that hypersensitivity to lights and sound affect the sleep cycle. Poor ability to calm themselves may affect children's bedtime routines. In addition, children may have a reduction in rapid eye movement sleep (Musumeci, Ferri, Elia, Dal Gracco, Scuderi, Stefanini, Castano, and Azan, 1995) and abnormal EEG patterns (Kluger, Bohm, Laub, and Waldenmaier, 1996).

Difficulties with falling or staying asleep seem to persist long past the time that other children are sleeping through the night.

Sensory defensiveness to light touch may cause even young children to arch their backs and resist being held. They may not like holding hands, tickling, and being cuddled. As they get older, they may also resist activities such as finger painting and working with certain textures. Deep pressure seems to be more acceptable, and even a comfort, to them.

Room lighting, sound levels, and distractions may all influence the attention and overall sensory state of persons with fragile X. These are some examples:

* ✳ Fluorescent lights, with their constant hum and flicker, may be poorly tolerated.

* ✳ Loud voices and lively discussions, loud music, gym whistles, fire alarms, and announcements over PA systems, may be too much for the easily overstimulated child.

* ✳ Visual distractions, such as bulletin boards and walls with every inch covered, may also cause anxiety and an unsettled state.

Hyperarousal may affect the development of speech and language, and early ear infections may distort auditory input, thus affecting language development (Braden, 2000b). Braden believes that the dysfunctional auditory system may contribute to an inconsistent filtering process that allows auditory input to seem either too loud or too muffled at times. Poor eye contact may also be the result of hyperarousal, and more repetitive, deviant language has been found when boys are forced to maintain eye contact (Belser and Sudhalter, 1995).

Behavioral outbursts may also be the effects of hyperarousal and anxiety. Self-regulation of mood and affect is often poor in persons with fragile X. New and strange routines, changes in schedules, and overwhelming lights, sounds, and crowds may all cause behavioral explosions. The antecedents to these outbursts may be seen in these ways:

* ✳ reddening of the face

* ✳ increased hand flapping

* ✳ pacing

* ✳ other physical signs of overstimulation.

This area will be explored more thoroughly in Chapter 6: Behavioral and Emotional Issues.

Self-help skills are another area that may be affected by hyperarousal and sensory overload. Personal hygiene may be difficult, as some children resist the stimulation of bathing, showering, brushing hair, brushing teeth, and later, shaving. Certain textures of clothing and tags may be disturbing, and soft, natural fabrics, with tags cut out, are often preferred.

Certain textures of clothing and tags may be disturbing, and soft, natural fabrics, with tags cut out, are often preferred.

Hypoarousal

There are others areas in which the child with fragile X does not seem to receive enough stimulus feedback. Self-stimulation, in the form of chewing on fingers, clothing, toys, or other items, seems to give boys with fragile X some input that they need. The need to smell or taste items may also be a reaction to a deficiency in feedback from those senses. Boys with fragile X are sometimes seen to sniff at items in order to arouse their sense of smell. Smell provides much information for these children, but they may move into others' personal space in order to better smell them and thus violate social cues about both proximity and behavior.

Hand flapping when anxious or excited also seems to be used as a calming mechanism and may be due to hypoarousal. The hand flapping, self-biting, and chewing on clothing and toys may involve a need for more proprioceptive awareness, a way to increase the information to the brain. On the other hand, these behaviors may be ways to shut out overstimulation or simply to deal with anxiety. Calming strategies may be the most needed to reduce these activities.

Difficulties with eating may be caused by both oral motor weaknesses and lack of awareness of feelings in the mouth area. Infants may have difficulty nursing or drinking from bottles, due to low muscle tone combined with tactile defensiveness. Children with fragile X often stuff too much food in their mouths and then choke, as they do not seem to have the sensation that their mouths are full, and that they need to chew and swallow. Lack of oral feedback may result in a need to create an oral sensation (stimulating the vibration sensitive vestibular system) through chewing on both edible and inedible items.

Children with fragile X often have very particular preferences about foods and may be picky eaters. Soft foods, which are easy to chew, are often preferred; however, there is a need to encourage chewing on hard, crunchy foods to help with oral motor development.

Toilet training is often delayed, simply because of cognitive level and overall awareness. There may, however, be issues of lack of sensation, particularly from hypotonal sphincter muscles, that cause boys to fail to realize that they need to go to the bathroom (Braden, 2000b). They must also motor plan how to get to the bathroom and deal with the challenges of removing clothing in time to use the toilet successfully. Poor diets, due to picky eating, may also contribute to a lack of roughage and problems with soft, uncontrolled stools.

Problems in Self-Regulation

Modulation of mood and affect may be major areas of concern for boys with fragile X. Emotional lability can be caused by anxiety and sensory overload. Boys with fragile X may express extreme reluctance to go to events and carry out activities, even when they have looked forward to them. Problems in self-regulation affect a number of areas, including attention, calming, and control of emotions. It is often boys' behavioral outbursts that are of concern to school administrators in considering inclusive programs. These behavioral issues will be explored more in Chapter 6: Behavior and Emotional Issues.

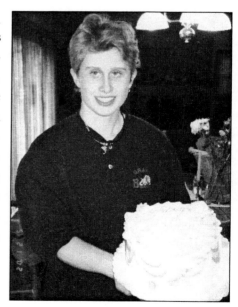

Visual-Motor Deficits

Motor coordination and planning issues may affect fine and gross motor activities. Both the vestibular system, the sense of gravity and one's movements in relation to it, governed by the inner ear, and the proprioceptive system, awareness of the body in space, may be compromised in children with fragile X (Saunders, 2001). Some children with fragile X do not have a good sense of themselves in space and walk into other people and objects. They may not have an appropriate awareness of distances and intrude into others' personal space.

Diagnosis of Sensory and Motor Issues

It is essential that boys and many girls with fragile X be assessed by an occupational therapist. An evaluation, as well as intervention, by an occupational therapist is vital, but all members of the educational team can be aware of and provide for sensory needs. Sensory processing, adaptive behavior, play, fine-motor skills, and visual-motor control can all be assessed through formal, standardized measures, criterion-referenced checklists, and observations.

The goal of diagnosis may be the formation of a "sensory diet" for children with fragile X. That involves finding the right combination of intensity, frequency, and duration of various sensory inputs to best help a child to be calm, alert, and responsive to learning. Much of the diagnosis may involve observing a child throughout a day, watching him cope with the rhythm of the day, and then suggesting interventions to provide appropriate sensory inputs.

Intervention for Sensory and Motor Issues

There are a number of areas that require goals and intervention for sensory and motor development. Sensory defensiveness and sensory overload, oral motor stimulation, self-help skills, and fine-motor skills all need to be addressed for many children with fragile X.

The chart on the following page displays some sources of possible sensory overload.

Sources of Possible Sensory Overload

Visual:
* ✳ Flickering or blinking lights
* ✳ Overcrowded bulletin board and walls
* ✳ Demands for eye contact

Auditory:
* ✳ High environmental noise volume
* ✳ Sudden noises
* ✳ High voice volumes (teachers and other children)
* ✳ Too much verbage (language overload)
* ✳ Emotional language (angry outbursts by teachers or other students)
* ✳ Negative language
* ✳ Demands for language output

Spatial:
* ✳ Crowding, close proximity

Routines:
* ✳ Changes in schedule
* ✳ Substitute teachers or aides

Calming Strategies

Team members may need to do careful observations in order to learn what is most calming for a child with fragile X. In order to design effective strategies for sensory overload, an analysis of the lighting, noise level, and decorations in classrooms and therapy rooms is essential. For some children, more natural lighting, rather than fluorescent bulbs, may be helpful. Rooms away from the noisiest parts of the school are preferable, and wall decorations may need to be kept to an uncluttered level. Teachers and therapists may need to be aware of their volume levels and tone, as children with fragile X may be very aware of and upset by loud or angry tones.

Deep Pressure

Therapeutic deep pressure may be calming for many boys with fragile X. The day might begin with wall pushups for everyone. Speech and language therapy sessions might be conducted with the occupational therapist, or at least with some deep pressure strategies for calming. These might include some deep pressure to the shoulders or making a "sandwich" with the boy's hand pressed between both of the therapist's. Some boys find it comforting to wear a weighted vest or arm bracelets in order to receive more pressure.

Deep Pressure Activities for Calming

Child activities:
* Wall push ups
* Chair push ups
* Sit in bean bag chair
* Rock in rocking chair
* Roll in blanket: "kid burrito"
* Lie between mats: "kid sandwich"
* Place palms together, push together
* Open and close hands
* Play with fidget toys

Teacher/therapist activities:
* Give bear hugs
* Apply deep pressure to shoulders
* Make "sandwich" with child's hand and press

Specialized clothing:
* Weighted vests
* Neoprene vests
* Lap "snakes"
* Pockets filled with heavy items
* Arm bands, wide and heavy watches

Heavy Work Activities

You might assign a boy with fragile X a variety of tasks that add to his sensory program. Heavy work can provide the sensory input needed to calm a child for a period of time. You might ask him to carry a stack of books back to the library, to lift and shelve boxes of toys, or to push chairs or a desk across a room. Sensory activities can be integrated into classroom time, with crawling on all fours through tunnels, crawling under tables and chairs, or performing an animal walk combined with a following directions activity. Physical games in gym or therapy, such as tug-of-war, throwing and catching a medicine ball, or hitting a punching bag, can provide strong sensory input.

Schedules

Pictured or written schedules are vital to classrooms and therapy rooms, as the need for routine is strong. Cues for transitions can be visual, so that the child can see each activity in sequence. They can also include advanced warnings, with such comments as, "Math time is starting at 10:00. You need to begin to clean up your table." Even if the child does not yet tell time or understand it, he can begin to hear the announcement and realize that the next class is imminent. Changes in schedule, 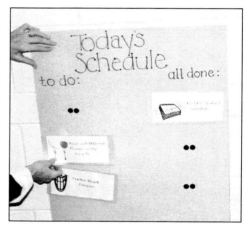 such as fire drills and field trips, must be dealt with according to the individual needs of the child. Schedules can include specific calming therapies, as well as be calming in and of themselves.

Managing Overstimulating Events

Some children cannot tolerate fire drills, assemblies, and field trips, and alternate plans may need to be made in these situations. Gradually building up a child's tolerance for change and for increased noise or crowds is an important goal, but it may take several years before a child can sit through an all-school assembly, particularly if it involves abstract information that is not easily understood (lectures on drug abuse) or loud, overwhelming programs (a band concert). The child with fragile X may need to be excused from such events, and later, with practice and role-playing, may attend such events but be allowed to leave with an aide, if necessary.

Sample Schedule:
Incorporating Sensory Activities in an Early Childhood Classroom

Morning routine:	Hang up jackets, put backpacks in cubbies, greet teachers and other students
Morning exercises:	Wall push ups
Circle time:	Calendar, weather, songs
Stations:	Speech/language, fine motor (OT), kitchen corner, block corner (complete 2 of 4)
Large group:	Story Circle
Gross Motor Activity	(integrated with story) incorporate deep pressure, swing, or bouncing on large ball
Snack:	Incorporate language with passing out napkins, cookies or crackers (aides can use deep pressure on shoulders, if necessary)
Stations:	Rotate through 2 more
Goodbye song:	Get jackets, backpacks

Signals

It is important to teach older children with fragile X to signal when they need a break. Such self-awareness and signals may be incorporated into IEP goals of older and higher functioning children, as they may be encouraged to use a signal, such as a "T" with their hands, to indicate that they need some time out.

Calming Spaces

Provide calming spaces in both classrooms and therapy rooms. Beanbag and rocking chairs provide firm, deep pressure, and rocking provides a way to self-stimulate and calm down. A corner with books on tape or music CDs with earphones can provide a respite area when a child is becoming agitated. Small pop-up tents, big boxes as "forts," study carrels, and small, walled-off cubicles in the classroom can also provide places to get away from the "crowd." At times, the staff may need to provide a blanket in which the child can roll up in a cocoon of comfort.

If a child is showing signs of becoming agitated, he may need to leave the classroom and find a calming space away from the entire class. If the school has a room equipped with therapeutic equipment, it might be used for a break on a swing, a time to bounce on a large ball, or a chance to sit and look at calming light patterns or watch a video.

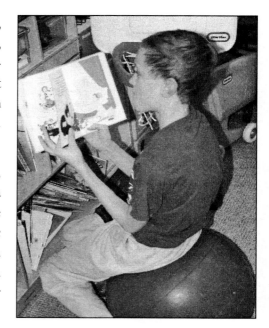

Oral Motor Goals

The development of oral motor skills is vital to most boys' goals. Such goals might be designed by speech-language pathologists or occupational therapists or a combined team of the two. Oral motor goals need to include both strengthening the oral musculature through exercises and building awareness through oral motor and speech sound activities. Oral motor goals include building tolerance for touch to the face and improving the ability to eat and drink (sucking from a straw, sensing the amount of food in the mouth, chewing and swallowing). There are numerous oral motor programs to use that include choices based upon individual goals and the amount of tolerance to touch that the child may have.

Self-Help Skills

Another very important area for occupational therapists and others to target is that of self-help skills. Dressing, grooming, toileting, eating, and doing daily chores require goals that fit the age and ability level of boys with fragile X.

✳ *Feeding Skills*

Goals for eating and drinking can initially be combined with oral motor strengthening goals to improve sucking and swallowing. Later, goals for eating may include more self-awareness. Verbal cues to alert the child to how much is in the mouth and the need to chew and then swallow, help awareness. Ground meats, chicken nuggets, and deli-style soft meats may be chewed more easily than roasted or fried meats. Setting a goal for eating a few bites of one new food item at a time is a way of slowly building up tolerance for a variety of textures and tastes.

✳ *Toileting*

Toilet training can be a particularly difficult challenge with boys who have fragile X syndrome. Overall cognitive level, in combination with a lack of sensory feedback, may cause boys to lack awareness of the need to use the toilet. Many of the classic toilet training methods that call for a consistent behavioral plan are appropriate. Diet is an important consideration in bowel training, as the limited foods that many boys eat might not include enough roughage and can cause loose stools.

✳ *Dressing*

Boys with fragile X often have delays in learning to dress, partially due to their cognitive levels and partially due to sensory issues. Here are some dressing tips:

- *Photos or other visual cues* (e.g., dressing/undressing in front of a mirror) help with memory for the items that need to be laid out each evening for the next day.

- *Attention must be paid to both comfortable items* (e.g. natural fabrics, tags cut from necks and waists) *and easy to wear clothing* (e.g., pants with gathered waists; tube socks, rather than those with heels; clip-on ties; loafers or slide type shoes).

- *Behavioral cues* for putting on jackets and flannel shirts (e.g., over the head) may be helpful.

- *Fine-motor skills* in buttoning, zipping, and tying should be included in occupational therapy goals. Backwards chaining and other behavioral cues can help with these tasks. Practice on actual clothing, with big buttons and zippers, may be more effective than dressing dolls and other small simulations of these activities.

✳ *At-Home Routines*

A number of self-help routines can be included in IEP goals that carry over to home activities. Parents may need help with ideas for baths, brushing hair and teeth, and bedtime routines.

Routines are very important for calming and working through the sensory issues involved in daily activities. Visual cues and schedules can be developed to help in these areas:

- *Bathing* (filling the tub, getting out favorite bath toys, shampooing hair, etc.)
- *Bedtime Sequence* (pictures of the child getting on pajamas, brushing teeth, being read a story, and getting into bed)

Occupational therapists may also suggest items and activities for sensory overload and calming, such as brushing the skin, deep pressure with towels and wash-cloths, and electric toothbrushes for deep stimulation.

Visual-Motor and Fine-Motor Goals

A final area for goal setting in the area of sensory development is that of visual-motor and fine-motor development. Many children with fragile X have visual strengths for memory of pictures, places, and whole words. Their fine-motor skills, however, may be hampered by lack of coordination, sensory defensiveness, and low muscle tone. Occupational therapists need to take leadership roles in designing goals for fine-motor development.

Hand strengthening, fine-motor, and flexibility goals may be set and pursued with a variety of activities:

- ✳ Work with clay, play dough, or theraputty to increase strength and flexibility.
- ✳ Hide small coins or other objects in the clay and have the child work to get them out.
- ✳ Use squeeze balls and sponges of varying densities for hand strengthening and as calming devices.
- ✳ Provide pegs, pegboards, and blocks to increase grasp and fine-motor control.

* Tie fine-motor activities to functional living skills and following directions by having children wring out a washcloth or towel, seal a plastic bag, or squirt a spray bottle filled with cleaning liquid.

* Introduce cooking by having children unscrew jar tops and open boxes.

* Practice dressing skills such as zipping, buttoning, and tying shoes.

Writing may be difficult, due to fine-motor issues, as well as to language and reading concerns. Writing should be encouraged and supported with these materials:
* stiff paper

* proper-sized pencils, markers, and crayons

* appropriate grips.

Writing stimuli should be uncluttered and simple, without overwhelming amounts of items on a page.

Teachers and therapists need to analyze whether a child works best with visual, auditory, or kinesthetic input before expecting visual-motor output (Johnson and Myklebust, 1967). Some children may require the motor pattern to be verbalized (e.g., "up, over"), while others may prefer to have their hands guided kinesthetically. Simple visual cues, such as color coding and boldfaced directions, can aid many children with fragile X in spelling and writing tasks. For example, a red "stop sign" may help a child with perseveration to stop going over and over a pattern.

Early work in writing letters, numbers, and shapes can be helped by the use of stencils and templates, simple tracing exercises, and dot-to-dots. Ultimately, many boys with fragile X may use word processing to more clearly write and space their words. Basic work on copying, simple writing, and writing signatures are also important for adult, functional living.

Conclusions

The various sensory issues discussed above pervade many aspects of the learning and development of children with fragile X. Programming for academic and behavioral growth must be designed with sensory issues in mind. Attention to learning environments can prevent a number of behavioral crises. If such issues are ignored, then maximum progress may not be seen in other areas of learning.

chapter 5

Speech and Language Development

One of the most significant and pervasive characteristics of children with fragile X syndrome is a disorder in speech and language. In fact, the lack of speech in young boys with fragile X is often the first indicator to parents that something is developmentally wrong with their child. In girls, many verbal skills may be strengths, but there are often significant needs in pragmatics, due to anxiety and poor social skills, which cause problems in conversational speech.

Causes of Speech and Language Disorders in Boys

There are a number of reasons for disorders in speech and language in boys with fragile X. Cognitive, physical, sensory, processing, and emotional issues all have an impact on speech and language development. There is a wide variation in the language skills of boys with fragile X, yet there is a remarkable similarity in the characteristics because of the underlying causes of their speech and language disorders.

Cognitive Effects

Overall cognitive level clearly has an effect on speech and language. The levels of receptive and expressive language that boys have are usually related to their nonverbal IQ score. There may be differences between their receptive and expressive language levels, and the better receptive score may be more likely to parallel the cognitive level.

Physical and Sensory Effects

There are a number of physical characteristics that cause speech and language disorders. Early recurrent episodes of otitis media often affect boys with fragile X, many before the age of six months (Schoenbrodt and Smith, 1995). Otitis media may be the result of hypotonia: low muscle tone that causes "floppy" Eustachian tubes. These ear infections may result in a fluctuating hearing loss, which contributes to an impairment of auditory perception, phonemic awareness, and articulation. Speech of boys with fragile X is often reported to be loud, which may be due to a minor hearing loss or poor processing of information. The effects of otitis media are influenced by the number and severity of the episodes of middle ear infection, the aggressiveness of treatment, and the effectiveness of that treatment.

Speech of boys with fragile X is often reported to be loud, which may be due to a minor hearing loss or poor processing of information.

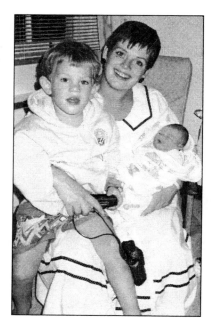

A high, arched palate is often seen in boys with fragile X, and there is a slightly higher incidence of cleft palate among this population (R. Hagerman, 2002b). Nasality and hearing may be affected as a result.

Oral sensory issues and hypotonia may cause numerous oral-motor problems. Boys with fragile X often have tactile defensiveness, particularly around their faces. Drooling, imprecise articulation, and difficulties with rapid sequences of speech have been reported (Rondal and Edwards, 1997). Families have also reported early problems with sucking and eating. Boys may have difficulties in chewing and swallowing to the degree that they stuff too much food in their mouths and choke. Swallowing issues may have to do with a lack of sensory feedback.

Cluttering, a fast and fluctuating rate of speech with repetitions of sounds, words, or phrases, may be related to hypotonia. Attention problems and hyperactivity also contribute to the rapid speech pattern.

Dyspraxic characteristics or motor planning problems, such as the following characterize many boys' speech production:

* dysfluencies
* poor production of sounds in words
* incorrect sequencing of sounds
* difficulties with polysyllabic words
* poor expressive language

Dyspraxia is often cited as the cause of some boys' lack of oral speech, thus necessitating the use of augmentative communication devices.

Voice quality of boys with fragile X is often reported to be hoarse and breathy, with odd pitch levels. Some speech-language pathologists notice a high, almost falsetto, pitch in older boys' speech, and others report a low pitch, perhaps due to low muscle tone.

Language Processing Problems

A number of language processing problems may affect speech and language development. Murphy and Abbeduto (2003) state that there is a dearth of data on underlying processing problems, as they specifically affect language, but there are a number of areas that seem to pervade the processing styles of boys with fragile X. Attention deficit disorders underlie many receptive language disorders in boys. Perceptual problems, such as auditory discrimination errors, often result from otitis media and the resulting mild hearing losses.

Problems in short-term memory, particularly for sequences and for non-meaningful input (e.g., strings of digits, random words), are often seen. Word retrieval seems to be an area of concern for many boys with fragile X, and a cluttered rhythm may result. Higher level auditory processing problems affect comprehension of spoken language, as word meanings, complex syntax structures, and abstract language are poorly understood.

Emotional/Behavioral Causes

A final area that is important to consider is that of the emotional and behavioral causes of speech and language disorders. Anxiety and hyperarousal are underlying factors that affect conversational skills, including turn taking, topic maintenance, perseveration, and eye contact. Attention deficit disorders also contribute to conversational problems, as social cues are not properly interpreted.

Characteristics of Speech-Language Disorders in Boys

Boys with fragile X have some unique, syndrome specific patterns of speech and language that differ from those of children with Down syndrome and other causes of mental retardation, although there are areas of similarity (Abbeduto and Hagerman, 1997; Abbeduto, Murphy, Cawthon, Richmond, Weissman, Karadottir, and O'Brien, 2003; Abbeduto, Pavetto, Kesin, Weissman, Karadottir, O'Brien, and Cawthon, 2001). In comparison studies, boys with Down syndrome were found to have more impairments in receptive and expressive language, as well as theory of mind, when compared to boys with fragile X syndrome. Perseverative speech was seen as the defining characteristic of the language of boys with fragile X by Abbeduto and Hagerman (1997). Roberts, Mirrett, and Burchinal (2001) and Roberts, Mirrett, Anderson, Burchinal, and Neebe (2002) found marked delays in language development, with a widening receptive-expressive gap over time, but they found great variability among individual children. The area of expressive speech and each of the language areas will be examined for defining characteristics.

Perseverative speech was seen as the defining characteristic of the language of boys with fragile X . . .

Non-speaking Boys

While many boys with fragile X speak their first words quite late, often in their second or third year, most do eventually use expressive speech. Some boys, however, have much better receptive skills than expressive, and do not use oral language. This may be due to dyspraxia, as their motor planning problems and oral motor weaknesses cause an inability to form sounds and words. For these boys, assessment of receptive knowledge must be conducted with special care, and appropriate augmentative devices must be found to adequately assess and enhance expressive capability.

Speech Production

The area of speech production is one that presents some of the unique features of fragile X. Boys with fragile X often have difficulty with both oral formulation and overall intelligibility. Their overall hyperarousal may affect their speech production, with a rapid, cluttered, poorly articulated quality. Articulation patterns are generally in keeping with their cognitive levels; however, their articulation may be affected by oral motor weaknesses and dyspraxia. Both vowels and consonants are reported as problematic for some children, with sound

Boys with fragile X often have difficulty with both oral formulation and overall intelligibility. Their overall hyperarousal may affect their speech production, with a rapid, cluttered, poorly articulated quality.

substitutions being common. In addition, sequencing of sounds in multisyllabic words is often hard, with transformations, such as *ephelant/elephant*. They often speak with a rapid, but dysrhythmic rate, and bursts of speech may be noted. They may rush through some phrases and sentences. Some may exhibit cluttered speech, with repeated syllables and whole words or phrases, but without the secondary characteristics of stuttering (Belser and Sudhalter, 1995, 2001).

Syntax Production

Receptive syntax development is generally in keeping with the nonverbal IQ scores of boys with fragile X. Murphy and Abbeduto (2003), in a review of a number of studies, found that the receptive syntax scores on the *Test of Auditory Comprehension of Language-Revised* (*TACL-R*) (Carrow-Woolfolk, 1985) were no different from those of younger, normally developing children who were matched for nonverbal IQ.

When looking at expressive syntax, Murphy and Abbeduto (2003) found a number of problems with the research. There are few studies of younger boys, and most research studies have small sample sizes, with varying age ranges of subjects in these studies. Most researchers use mean length of utterance (MLU) as their measure of expressive syntax, but they use a variety of language sampling techniques. Murphy and Abbeduto believe that the use of conversations for language sampling does not tax the child's expressive capabilities and may result in less than maximal output. Instead of relying solely on MLU, we may need to use a variety of language sampling techniques and aim for both typical and maximal syntax (see Wren, 1985, for language sampling techniques and rationales).

Most boys do learn to speak in whole sentences, although some remain at the level of short phrases. They may have particular syntax problems with question forms (e.g., "What it is?"), negatives, and pronoun usage. Some boys reverse pronouns or use their own names rather than "I" or "me" when talking about themselves (e.g., "Jack needs a nap"). The cluttering quality of boys' speech causes breakdowns in syntax, along with syllable repetition, false starts, and a rapid and irregular rate.

Semantics

Single word receptive vocabulary is generally seen as a relative strength for boys with fragile X, with single word vocabulary higher than comprehension of vocabulary in connected language. Boys may show an unexpectedly strong concrete vocabulary, especially in areas of personal interest (e.g., names of cars, animals) (Braden, 2000b). For example, a boy who is interested in animals may know specific words such as *primate* and *reptile* that are well above his tested expressive vocabulary. Words seem to be learned best in contextual situations, which is why boys often pick up words from books, TV shows, and videos.

Words seem to be learned best in contextual situations, which is why boys often pick up words from books, TV shows, and videos.

Murphy and Abbeduto (2003) report that the data are inconsistent as to whether achievement in lexical domains keeps pace with, exceeds, or lags behind nonlinguistic cognitive levels or other language domains. They see the receptive-expressive gap growing with age, but state that there are not enough longitudinal data on vocabulary growth. They believe that the IQ decline, which was discussed in Chapter 3: Cognitive Development, may reflect a slowed rate of cognitive development, closely tied to that of lexical development. As vocabulary assessment of older children includes more multiple meaning words and more abstract vocabulary, vocabulary scores may decrease on standardized tests. This does not mean that boys are losing vocabulary, but that their vocabulary development is not keeping pace with that of their peers.

Both receptive and expressive vocabulary knowledge and use are affected by the concrete-abstract nature of the vocabulary. As with other children who have language disorders, the understanding of multiple meaning words, more abstract terms, idioms, metaphors, and similes poses great difficulties for children with cognitive weaknesses due to fragile X.

Pragmatics

Pragmatics, the area of communication that governs conversation, is often the major area of difficulty for boys with fragile X. While the areas of syntax and semantics present themselves as areas of language delay, the broader area of pragmatics is one of considerable language disorder. The areas of language, socialization, and cognition all intersect to limit the child's acquisition of pragmatic skills.

Social anxiety and hyperarousal cause poor eye contact, especially in older boys and men. Poor eye contact is manifested in a number of different kinds of tasks. With their poor eye contact and poor nonverbal awareness, males with fragile X may miss important cues provided by facial expressions (e.g. happy, sad, angry), as well as tone of voice. The high level of arousal causes a trade-off between the intense discomfort of the direct gaze and the ability to offer appropriate language. Some speech-language pathologists have chosen not to emphasize more than fleeting eye contact, as it may cause the boy or man with fragile X to trade expressive language for eye contact.

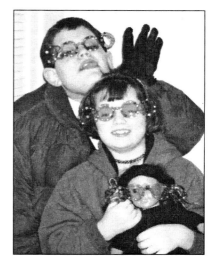

The "fragile X handshake" is seen when a boy or man literally turns his body away and averts his gaze, while extending his hand in greeting.

As many boys and men want to be friendly, they make social attempts with inappropriate skills. The "fragile X handshake" is seen when a boy or man literally turns his body away and averts his gaze, while extending his hand in greeting. This might be an area where speech-language pathologists want to work on some level of eye contact for more appropriate social interactions.

Topic maintenance and turn taking are often poor, affected by anxiety, in addition to both attention and comprehension issues. Boys do not always make their intentions clear to others and don't take steps to get additional information. Murphy and Abbeduto (2003) believe that this is a result of the challenges of interpersonal understanding and attention, rather than a purely language challenge. Direct questioning of boys seems to result in a high level of anxiety to the degree that their answers may be off topic, even when they are following the conversation. This is a major area for intervention, and a speech-language pathologist can provide structured cues for conversation.

Perseverative language is perhaps the unique and defining characteristic of fragile X syndrome (Abbeduto and Hagerman, 1997). There is an especially high rate of self-repetitions and off-topic or tangential utterances in the conversation of boys with fragile X. Children may ask the same question over and over, even after it has been answered several times. When the question is turned back to them, they can often show that they know the answer.

Those boys with fragile X who exhibit autistic-like characteristics, but who do not meet all the diagnostic criteria for autism, usually have much repetitive, perseverative language, but not as much echolalia as boys with autism. Verbal imitation and modeling are powerful strengths for many boys with fragile X. They frequently learn and use automatic phrases or whole chunks of information gleaned from familiar settings. While these phrases may be used appropriately in some settings, they have the quality of delayed echolalia, often sounding like verbatim quotes from videos and TV shows (Harris-Schmidt and Fast, 1998). They may also repeat whole strings of swear words, indicating their good ability to model their peers!

Murphy and Abbeduto (2003) believe that three different possible causes for the presence of so much perseverative language need to be explored:

1. *arousal state*, as explored by Belser and Sudhalter (2001)

2. *abnormalities in the frontal lobe*, resulting in executive function weaknesses (the inability to inhibit high strength or previously activated responses)

3. *limited expressive language*, with a need for more processing time.

Determination of the cause of a child's perseverative language could give us information about how to intervene in this important area.

Literacy Learning

While most boys with fragile X have reading levels in keeping with their overall cognitive levels, there are some particular characteristics of their reading patterns that seem to be unique:

* They seem to read by a whole word method, using their visual strengths for whole word memorization.

* Phonemic awareness, including the analysis and synthesis of words by phonics methods, is more difficult for most (Johnson-Glenberg, 2003).

* Some boys are described as hyperlexic — early readers who "word call," but don't have the comprehension to match their visual recognition skills (Harris-Schmidt and Fast, 1998).

Written language, the highest form of language use, is generally in keeping with cognitive level and reading skills. Whole word spelling may be an area of relative strength, with difficulties in oral formulation and sequencing of ideas. Some difficulties in fine-motor areas cause additional problems in written language.

Characteristics of Speech and Language Disorders in Girls

Areas of Strength

There are far fewer studies of girls' language, but some descriptions are emerging from the research. As a group, girls with fragile X syndrome have higher language levels overall than boys. Their verbal IQs, vocabulary, and syntax often fall in the average range, even if other cognitive and language areas are lower. When compared to a group of boys with fragile X, matched for overall IQ, girls were noted to have most of the same patterns as boys, although their expressive syntax levels (based up MLUs) were higher. (Abbeduto, Murphy, Cawthon, Richmond, Weissman, Karadottir, and Obrien, 2003; Murphy and Abbeduto, 2003). Strengths are seen in many areas of concrete language learning. Girls are often good readers and have adequate spelling and writing skills, as opposed to their weaknesses in mathematics.

Areas of Weakness

An area of weakness for girls and women with fragile X, even those who test in the normal range of intelligence, is that of pragmatics. Anxiety issues seem to underlie many areas of weakness in conversations. Poor social awareness, tangential speech, organizational problems, and poor eye gaze may all be present in interactive language situations. Some have run-on, disorganized speaking styles, with flighty attention to topic.

An area of weakness for girls and women with fragile X, even those who test in the normal range of intelligence, is that of pragmatics.

Some of their pragmatic disorders are related to broader nonverbal learning disabilities. These include problems in executive functioning, or meta-awareness in planning and monitoring their actions; visual-spatial processing; and mathematics. Difficulties with nonverbal processing can cause breakdowns in the understanding of cues in conversation, such as tone (sarcasm, humor), facial expressions, and volume.

Some girls also have difficulty with auditory memory for sequences, which causes problems in following multiple directions. They also may have difficulty with more abstract language, and do better when taught expository information in a narrative manner, such as history lessons through the stories of the people who were there instead of textbook presentations of facts, dates, and events.

Hagerman, Hills, Scharfenaker, and Lewis (1999) have studied some cases of girls with selective mutism. Extremely high levels of anxiety, panic attacks, shyness, and tactile defensiveness were found in the girls who had selective mutism. These girls responded well to medication, such that they were able to overcome the mutism. Interestingly, Hagerman et al. (1999) found that girls who had ADHD (approximately 35% of the girls in their study) did not show the high levels of social anxiety, and none of those had selective mutism. They conclude that girls with ADHD may be somehow protected from significant social anxiety.

Speech and Language Assessment

Speech and language assessment by a speech-language pathologist is essential for all children with fragile X syndrome. Whether children are at the early intervention or the adolescent level, diagnosis and intervention by a speech-language pathologist are vital. Diagnosis must be carried out with other individuals on a multi-disciplinary team and with all of the contributing areas to speech and language disorders in mind: cognitive, sensory, and emotional/behavioral.

Diagnosis of speech-language disorders needs to include those components that are often mentioned in the characteristics descriptions. A thorough audiological examination, particularly in light of the high incidence of middle ear pathology, should precede any speech-language assessment. The effects of myringotomies (the placement of tubes in the ears) or of prophylactic antibiotics, designed to prevent ear infections, can make a great difference in speech and language test results.

A thorough oral-motor exam is also essential, but it may be difficult to carry out with the level of oral/tactile defensiveness that many children with fragile X have. Teaming with an occupational therapist can provide the necessary joint expertise to complete the exam. Examination of the palate, tongue movement and strength, lip closure and strength, sucking, and swallowing can lead to intervention goals in the areas of speech and swallowing. If the child is resistant to touch around the face, some of the assessment may need to be done initially by observation of eating, drinking, and speech.

There are many standardized, norm-referenced tests that can be given in the areas of vocabulary, syntax, morphology, and articulation/phonology. It is important to keep in mind, when administering formal tests, that the contributing factors of anxiety, difficulty with direct questioning, attention deficit disorders, and dislike of changes in routine may cause scores to be minimal estimates. Consider areas of language processing while analyzing test results. Richard (2001) provides a number of assessment ideas for language processing that might be kept in mind when administering standardized tests, in addition to ideas for informal checklists and activities.

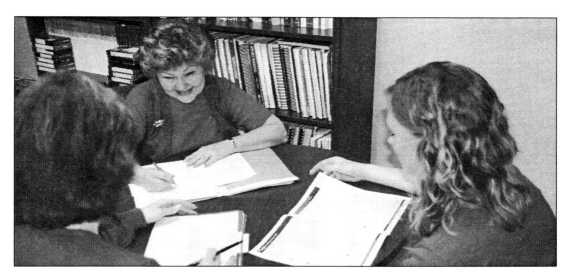

While some researchers see a plateau in scores (Fisch, Holden, Carpenter, Howard-Peebles, Maddalena, Pandya, and Nance, 1999) of people with fragile X, most believe that progress continues across the age span (Roberts, Mirrett, and Burchinal, 2001), and that standardized tests do not always measure the achievements that are seen outside of the test arena (Braden, 2000b).

A variety of test adaptations need to be made for children who are non-speaking. Thorough measures of receptive skills, coupled with informal expressive measures, the use of gestures, pictures, and/or signs provide the best measures of capability of non-speaking children. Speech-language pathologists may gain knowledge about comprehension and thinking skills by observing a psychologist administering a measure of nonverbal intelligence.

Portfolios, language samples, and criterion referenced tests can be used in place of or in addition to standardized tests. Portfolios, which include materials used in thematic language units that display evidence of vocabulary learning, and language samples measuring syntax progress are important alternative assessment tools. Criterion referenced tests, which simply measure an individual child's progress, may be used at various times during the year to assess growth in specific skills.

Equally important in the speech and language assessment, is the use of observations and checklists to evaluate attention deficit disorder, processing, and autism. A variety of observers can be asked to fill out measures that would lead to a referral for testing by a pediatric neurologist for attention deficit disorder or to an autism specialist.

Assessment is clearly an ongoing process with children who have fragile X syndrome. A diagnostic teaching model may provide the best insights and results, as assessment is included as part of ongoing therapy. Rather than only assessing when benchmarks are due or IEPs are to be updated, regular, ongoing assessment helps us see real progress with meaningful, appropriate tasks.

Intervention for Speech-Language Disorders

Guiding Principles

Intervention in the areas of speech and language is essential for all children with fragile X syndrome across the age span. Goals and intervention should be developed in conjunction with other professionals on the IFSP or IEP team. Several effective models for SLP/OT programming have shown success in combining calming strategies (e.g., deep pressure, breathing, muscle relaxation) with language activities (Stackhouse and Scharfenaker, 2002). Language programming in the special education or regular education classroom may be the most successful intervention strategy, as pragmatic/conversational language is often the focus. Speech-language pathologists often find themselves in new situations when working with a child with fragile X. The SLP may be putting on her sneakers and heading for the playground to work on social skills, eating lunch with the child to facilitate appropriate social skills with peers during the informal setting of the lunchroom, or having lunch with a small group of children to explain the special needs of a child with fragile X to classmates.

Language programming in the special education or regular education classroom may be the most successful intervention strategy, as pragmatic/conversational language is often the focus.

As much as possible, children with fragile X need to be with their peers in regular education, in order to model appropriate language and play skills. For some children with significant behavioral and academic issues, the regular education classroom may not be appropriate, but there are ways to do some "reverse mainstreaming" and have peers from regular education come into the special education room for activities.

Other areas that need to be kept in mind throughout planning for speech and language goals and intervention include the following:

* visual cues (pictures, logos, words, signs)
* visual schedules
* need for routine
* planning for transitions and changes in routine
* calming activities
* calming spaces

Areas for Intervention

* *Language Processing*
  A number of processing areas affect language learning and need to be kept in mind when designing therapy.

  * Attention
    With the underlying attention problems that many children with fragile X have, a thorough diagnosis and medical and behavioral intervention are necessary (see Chapter 6: Behavior and Emotional Issues). The establishment of a calm, quiet atmosphere can be helpful for addressing attention problems. Speech-language pathologists need to establish areas that are not overwhelming and distracting visually, are quiet, and provide some calming spaces and activities (e.g., bean bag chairs with books or music on tapes). Attention and perception may also be aided by the use of earphones and FM amplification systems. If the SLP is conducting group lessons, she can wear a small microphone in order to help the child with fragile X to focus on her voice. The establishment of routines can also help with attention, as well as anxiety and hyperarousal. The child with fragile X may be able to focus better knowing how many activities are planned and how to check each one off in a schedule format.

  * Perception/Auditory Discrimination
    SLPs need to conduct perception checks when presenting auditory information to be sure the child understood the proper word. They need to describe the words where possible or use them in sentences to check understanding. Visual cues, such as objects, signs, pictures, and later words, can help assure accurate auditory perception.

- Short-term Memory
  There are a variety of strategies that can address short-term memory problems. Simple attention strategies can help the SLP or teacher know that the child heard the directions (e.g., "Repeat what I just told you to do"). Question-answer-question formats (e.g., "What kind of animal is a zebra? It's a mammal. What kind of animal is a zebra?") allow the therapist to state, repeat, and check that information has been received. Visual cueing is vital to aid memory. Visualization strategies help the child remember auditory information. For instance, in making a list of items to buy for a cooking project, the SLP can have the child visualize the aisles in the store and repeat the items that need to be purchased. Visual cues, such as semantic networks and other graphic organizers, are effective in aiding memory and comprehension of stories and expository information. Mneumonic devices, such as associations, can help with memory for names and other factual information. Once a child with fragile X stores information in memory, long-term memory seems to be a relative strength, so that information can be used purposefully.

- Higher Level Language Processing
  Higher level language processing, at the levels of symbolization and conceptualization relates to the understanding of language and integration of ideas. Most clinicians recommend functional, meaningful lessons that tie into areas of interest and/or applications for the child with fragile X. While a child with fragile X may be able to memorize isolated bits of information, those bits will not be understood unless they are tied to concrete, meaningful applications.

* *Comprehension*
  Comprehension of language becomes intertwined with anxiety issues. Direct questioning may not be the best means by which to work on comprehension. Strategies that use oral "fill in the blank" or multiple choice formats may be much more successful. For instance, a teacher or therapist might say, "First we put the cake mix in the _____" instead of, "What did we put the cake mix in?" or "What did we do first?" These types of presentations eliminate the confusion with *Wh-* questions that the child may not understand.

✳ *Oral Motor*

Boys with fragile X syndrome often present an interesting contrast in oral motor needs. They have a marked need for self-stimulation in the mouth area and often chew on their fingers, hands, clothing, toys, and crayons. On the other hand, they may have an intolerance for the touch of others around their faces and mouths, particularly light, feathery touches. They have a hypersensitivity to the tactile stimulation of others, but a hyposensitivity to their own chewing and swallowing needs (stuffing too much food in their mouths without realizing it, for example). Oral motor therapy is a primary goal for most boys with fragile X syndrome.

Oral motor therapy can be designed with two different, but related, goals:

1. activities to strengthen the oral musculature

2. awareness activities of placements (e.g. of tongue, lips, and teeth) that foster clearer articulation

Goals might include such areas as:

✳ decrease defensiveness around mouth area

✳ decrease need for self-stimulation (including chewing on self, clothing, toys)

✳ increase strength in oral musculature

✳ increase tolerance for textures in foods

✳ increase self-awareness of chewing and swallowing issues

✳ increase self-awareness of positions of tongue, lips, and teeth for formation of various sounds

Therapists need to provide items for chewing that can replace inappropriate items such as the child's skin or clothing. Chewy candies, such as fruit snacks or licorice, and sour candies can provide a good amount of sensory input. Hard, crunchy items, such as carrots, apple slices, and toasted bagels can also serve the same need. Some therapists provide chewy tubing, such as aquarium tubing, in lengths that cannot be choked. A tube may be used as a necklace that the child can reach for and chew when nervous or overstimulated.

Strengthening of the oral musculature can be fostered with bubble blowing, whistle blowing, and work with straws. Sucking from a straw may be difficult for a child with weak oral musculature. Therapists should begin with larger, shorter straws (not the thin type, as in juice boxes), and may begin by tipping the straw up for the child. Work with oral motor strengthening can then be tied to speech goals, such as lip strengthening in blowing bubbles and in saying sounds, such as /p/, /b/, and /m/.

Cues for chewing and swallowing may need to be provided. Helping the child to monitor how much he has put in his mouth may be vital in order to help with both safe and appropriate eating.

✳ *Articulation/Phonology*

Poor oral motor control, coupled with motor planning problems, such as sequencing sounds, results in poor intelligibility for many boys. Poor intelligibility of some boys' speech is also a result of their fast rate and repetitious, cluttered speaking.

Some boys are diagnosed with dyspraxia of speech, which means the child has difficulty with the purposeful, voluntary movement sequences for speech when there is no paralysis of the oral musculature. When asked to place their tongues, teeth, or lips in certain positions, the children with dyspraxia cannot voluntarily do so. Their connected speech is more unintelligible than their single word productions, with a variety of inconsistent errors. Sequencing of sounds is especially difficult, and there may be multiple speech sound errors (Yorkston, Beukelman, Strand, and Bell, 1999). Specific therapy goals and strategies that are centered on motor speech disorders need to be addressed for such children. These children may not respond to typical articulation therapy, and their patterns are not those of children with phonological disorders.

For children with verbal motor planning problems, a motor planning therapy approach needs to address these areas:

- emphasis on movement patterns in syllables, moving from the simplest (one syllable words such as "pop") to the more complex
- drill on simple and most visible sounds
- use of intensive, paired auditory and visual stimuli
- imitation of sustained vowels and consonants
- production of sound combinations

- focus on movement performance drill

- use of repetitive production and intensive, systematic drill

- use of decreased rate

- use of carrier phrases

- use of stress, intonation, and rhythm

- enhancement of kinesthetic awareness

- establishment and practice of core vocabulary
  (www.apraxia-kids.org/definitions/litrev; Yorkston et al., 1999)

Whether or not boys are diagnosed with motor speech disorders, it is often helpful to work with slowing the rate and rhythm of speech to improve intelligibility. Songs, poems, and choral work help with the flow of speech. Strategies that are used for stuttering, such as slow, easy speech, are appropriate for boys with cluttering issues.

✳ *Augmentative and Alternative Communication*

Augmentative and alternative communication (AAC) allows for development of expressive language for those who are nonverbal and can serve as a bridge to spoken language. Augmentative communication is defined as an approach that is in addition to natural speech and/or handwriting, while alternative communication refers to an approach that is a substitute for natural speech or handwriting (Senner, 2002). Research literature has shown that the use of AAC does not inhibit speech development; rather, it actually facilitates the development of speech (Senner, 2002). It provides a way for a nonverbal child to express himself and reduces communicative frustration.

Research literature has shown that the use of AAC does not inhibit speech development; rather, it actually facilitates the development of speech.

AAC can accompany oral language, enabling the child to have both auditory and visual input through signs, picture boards, and/or computerized interactive devices. Children can learn some natural or universal gestures, such as shrugs, points, and miming or they can use visual "props" to help them "tell" their families about an event. For example, a child might show a family member a leaf from a nature field trip or the program from a chorus concert (Yorkston et al., 1999).

The field of computerized, augmentative devices is expanding rapidly, and speech-language pathologists need to know how to best access and use these devices with nonverbal children. It is beyond the scope of this chapter to review augmentative communication in depth, but it is an important area for speech-language pathologists and special educators to explore when expressive communication is lagging far behind receptive.

✳ *Syntax*

Goals in the area of syntax may be designed to increase both length and complexity of phrases and sentences. Keeping in mind the processing weaknesses in attention, short-term memory, and sequencing, goals can be aimed at attention to and memory for longer utterances. Receptive understanding of more complex phrases and sentences and expressive use of them can be targets.

Visual cues are an excellent way to aid auditory learning:
- Simple hand signs enhance comprehension of oral directions.
- Flannel boards, sentence pockets, and computer programs add visual and hands-on elements to syntax work.
- Pictured sentence cards illustrate words, such as adjectives and adverbs, and provide necessary cues.
- Scrambled sentences, with words on separate cards, help children understand questions versus statements and foster understanding.
- Fill-in-the-blank sentences help children add descriptive words to their vocabulary and finish prepositional phrases.

Traditional syntax strategies, such as modeling, expansion, and parallel talk are very appropriate for children with fragile X.

Therapists may control speech rate and work with slowed speech in order to improve sequencing in sentences. It's important to emphasize omitted words and words out of order to help with attention to smaller, function words (e.g. "What IS this?" when working to change, "What this is?").

Therapists and teachers may be able to use the long, memorized phrases that some children with fragile X have stored in long-term memory (delayed echolalia) as learning tools. These phrases can be altered slightly, through visual cues, such as word or picture cards, to encourage new meanings. For example, a phrase such as, "Part of your complete breakfast" from an advertisement can be altered and expanded with various terms, such as, "Toast is 'part of your complete breakfast,'" or "Cereal is 'part of your complete breakfast.'"

Work with question formation is a challenge for many children who have language disorders, and may be especially difficult for children with both cognitive weaknesses and autistic-like symptoms. When asked to form a question to ask another person, children with fragile X may need a good deal of modeling and visual cues for the *Wh-* words. The simpler forms, such as *what* and *who* can be incorporated into thematic units and literacy activities. It may be best to begin with asking and answering questions with concrete, one-word answers. Gradually, students can be encouraged to make up questions about a story or activity, given the *Wh-* word cues.

Work with question formation is a challenge for many children who have language disorders, and may be especially difficult for children with both cognitive weaknesses and autistic-like symptoms.

✳ *Semantics*

Receptive vocabulary is a relative strength for many boys with fragile X, and it is important to be aware that more understanding may be taking place than the child is able to express. Clearly, the goals for semantics must be designed with the cognitive level of the child in mind, but based upon the philosophy that language can lead cognition (as explained by Vygotsky, 1957), work with semantic goals should not be abandoned because of a child's lower cognitive ability.

Goals should center around expansion of vocabulary and the semantic relations among terms that are of special interest to the child. Language units should start with basic object levels and move from the most typical examples to more peripheral, and include superordinates, subordinates, and features. For instance, units on animals might move from names and descriptions of familiar, typical animals within a category (lions, tigers, monkeys as jungle animals), to less typical or familiar jungle animals (macaw, toucan) to animal categories (mammals, birds, reptiles), subordinate categories (types of monkeys) and their features (fur). Visual cues, such as real animals, stuffed animals, pictures, and videos should always accompany language units. Acting out words and their use in sentences can bring a visual, nonverbal cue to the storage of the word in memory. The child might act out a "fierce" lion or a "playful" monkey.

When moving from areas of high interest to other areas that need to be covered in the curriculum, it is important to continue to use meaningful materials to expand meanings and work towards some levels of abstraction. Girls and higher functioning boys may have semantic goals in the areas of literature, science, and social studies. SLPs can work with classroom teachers and pre-teach specific vocabulary before various units begin. Vocabulary work should always include visual cues and meaningful connections. For example, maps, map puzzles, and souvenirs from travels might be used to explain geography.

✻ *Pragmatics*
Addressing pragmatics, or conversational skills, is the primary need in nearly all boys and many girls with fragile X. For many children with fragile X, reduction of anxiety and hyperarousal is integral to the success of pragmatic therapy (Sudhalter, 2002). Specific goals might focus upon the following:

- perseveration
- topic maintenance
- tangential comments
- self-talk
- echolalia
- eye contact

Structured verbal rehearsal in role-plays, scripted situations, and guided conversations can help lower anxiety levels and lead to success in more spontaneous situations. Job tasks and other functional language activities are essential parts of the IEP for most children with fragile X and can be integrated as success in highly structured, small group activities has been achieved.

Role-plays and verbal rehearsal can address pragmatic needs and improve functional language. The following page illustrates a role-play of a job task that can be incorporated into the daily schedule of a boy with fragile X.

Role-Play Example

Job:
* Pick up all attendance lists outside fifth grade classrooms.
* Take the lists to the office and give them to school secretary.

Oral language goal:
* Say, "Mrs. Sullivan, here is the attendance." When she says, "Thank you," answer, "You're welcome."

Paralinguistic goal:
* Establish at least fleeting eye contact.

Sensory motor/behavioral:
* Walk with arms at sides (no flapping) and quietly (no self-talk).

Strategies to achieve such a goal would include rehearsal of the activity and visual cues, such as a sign for, "Quiet mouth." Practice walking down the hall might include a teacher to cue for "arms at sides." Rate and rhythm, clarity of articulation, and appropriate voice can all be incorporated into the functional language activity.

Conversational goals aimed at an appropriate level for the child involve working on initiating conversation, topic maintenance, and controlling tangential comments and perseveration. SLPs may start with simple greetings and responses, as well as courtesies (e.g., "How are you?" "Fine, how are you?"). These may be built up to structured group conversations, which are highly scripted at first. Simple turn-taking around such topics as what classmates did over the weekend or what they brought for lunch can be scripted and gradually expanded to include follow-up questions and comments. Braden's (2002b) four level social skills program involves simple turn taking (with objects and games) with an adult in level one and gradually building up to verbal exchanges with both adults and peers. The adult initially models and provides scripts for imitation and gradually moves back to facilitate interaction between two students, with prompts and scripting.

Within any conversational goals, strategies may be needed to control perseveration (e.g., turning the question back to the child after a questions with a known answer has been asked over and over, providing cues that a topic is now over). In the same way, tangential comments should be controlled through cues such as, "We're talking about Matt's weekend now, not the Power Rangers. Can you ask Matt one questions about his weekend?"

Social interactions may need to be prompted with specific games such as, "Find a friend who _____," in which the student must ask specific interview questions about favorite colors, activities, and interests. SLPs may also find they are spending IEP minutes on the playground or in the lunchroom. They may be helping children who have fragile X learn how to ask to join a game or to sit at a group lunch table.

Social stories, based upon the work of Carol Gray (1995) have proven to be very successful with children who have a number of social, behavioral, and pragmatic problems. Social stories may be designed to help a child through a situation in which his or her behavior has been inappropriate or in which the teacher or SLP

Social Skills Story Example

My friends like to play with the four square balls at recess.

Sometimes, I start to take the balls and put them in the bag to take back into school.

My friends get upset when I take their ball away in the middle of the game.

I will try to wait until the recess teacher blows the whistle and tells me to pick up all the balls.

Then, my friends will be happy that they got to finish their game.

---

wants the child to understand the dynamics of a situation better. Social stories are scripted and allow the child to read and re-read or hear a story read many times and in several settings. Social stories often have descriptive and reflective sentences, and include a sentence that begins with an "I will try . . ." statement.

A variation of the social story concept has been developed by Gagnon (2001), which uses a child's favorite fictional characters as the motivators. Using her *Power Cards* concept, the speech-language pathologist or teacher might name a TV character who knows the importance of the behavior that the child is working on and encourages the child to do it.

Eye contact, while a significant problem for many boys and some girls with fragile X, may not be an appropriate area for pragmatic goals. Researchers have found that language tends to decrease when eye contact is forced. The classic "Look at me" command may cause such hyper-arousal in the child with fragile X that language goals and strategies may become secondary to dealing with the need to look at the conversational partner. Joint attention, with the child and therapist or teacher seated at a 90-degree angle, may be more appropriate than face-to-face sessions.

Researchers have found that language tends to decrease when eye contact is forced.

It may be appropriate to work with "fleeting" eye contact for greetings and closings and as strategies to get someone's attention. Games, such as "stare down" contests, with hands palm to palm, or having two children alternate the spelling of a word, can be used to foster longer periods of eye contact. Gradually, children with fragile X seem to become more comfortable with sustained eye contact, especially with those with whom they are familiar.

✳ *Language Literacy Issues*
Goals in the area of language also extend into reading and writing goals. Reading may be used both as a visual strategy to aid language and behavior (e.g., with written schedules, lists of activities, scripts, and social stories), and language goals may be incorporated into reading goals and activities. Some boys with fragile X are described as hyperlexic. They learn to recognize whole words at an early age, but don't always have the comprehension to match their word recognition skills.

Generally, reading strengths are seen in simultaneous processing of whole words. Weaknesses in phonemic processing and sequencing cause a phonics approach to be less successful. Whole word approaches may include pictures or logos. Braden's (1989) *Logo Reading System* is based upon using familiar signs and shapes in order to build up a sight vocabulary. She might begin with a logo, such as Pizza Hut or Burger King and gradually move the familiar word (e.g. *king*) into word families, other contexts, and sentences. Rebus methods utilize pictures integrated with simple words to accomplish growing sight recognition.

For more advanced readers, language can be integrated into reading comprehension activities through pre-teaching vocabulary and concepts. In inclusive classrooms, speech-language pathologists may pre-teach the vocabulary in the classroom curriculum unit and break down concepts into simpler terms. Narratives can be used to teach expository concepts, and activities such as acting out stories, drawing pictures, and seeing videos are very helpful.

Writing skills may be hampered by fine motor, as well as cognitive and language weaknesses. Goals and activities for fine-motor control may center around letter and word formation, spacing, and spelling. For some children, the fine-motor act is so difficult that alternatives to writing may need to be found. Saunders (2001) suggests the use of a word processor for some written language activities, worksheets with single words to be filled in or circled, and alternative ways to show knowledge, such as dictation into a tape recorder, oral rather than written responses, and the acceptance of pictures rather than sentences. She states that "a little and often" is the best way to ensure written success. For such children, goals may simply be to be able to fill in a form, write a signature, and make a list.

Spelling may be an area of relative strength, due to strengths in visual simultaneous processing. Spelling words may be taught in word families to show visual similarities, and strategies such as scrambled words and fill-in-the-blanks may help with visual recognition. With older and higher functioning children, syllables and meaningful morphemes may be used to expand spelling words (e.g., *dance, dancing, dancer*).

For other children, written language goals also need to include ideation and generation of language. Structured written language, with visual cues, can help children form complete sentences and paragraphs. Written cues, such as sentence starters and transition words, can control perseverative thoughts and provide links for ideas. Guided writing can be used with students to stimulate a flow of ideas and the idea that one thought connects to another to build a paragraph. This can be done using some of the core content vocabulary and spelling words. The areas of reading and written language will be expanded upon in Chapter 8: Academic Intervention.

Conclusions

The areas of speech and language present significant challenges for most boys and many girls with fragile X syndrome. Receptive and expressive language and the literacy areas of reading and writing are all appropriate for intervention. An integrated plan that includes knowledge of cognitive, sensory, and emotional needs can be successful in helping these children make significant gains. Speech and language development does not end at the elementary years. Rather, speech and language intervention is a vital area for intervention from infancy through adulthood.

chapter 6

Behavioral and Emotional Issues

Behavioral and emotional issues affecting children with fragile X syndrome:

common to boys

✳ behavioral outbursts

✳ attention deficit/hyperactivity disorders

✳ anxiety

✳ autistic-like characteristics

common to girls

✳ anxiety

✳ anxiety accompanied by depression

✳ attention deficit-hyperactivity disorders of the predominantly inattentive type (ADHD-I)

A significant number of behavioral and emotional issues affect both boys and girls with fragile X syndrome. Clearly, not all behaviors are a result of fragile X syndrome, yet there are commonalities among those of many children with the syndrome. Behavioral outbursts, attention deficit/hyperactivity disorders (ADHD), and anxiety, along with autistic-like characteristics, are common to many boys with fragile X. Girls with fragile X often have significant issues with anxiety — sometimes accompanied by depression — and may have attention deficit/hyperactivity disorders of the predominantly inattentive type (ADHD-I). These areas of behavioral and emotional development are ones that require an integrated plan of medical, behavioral, and therapeutic response.

Behavioral Characteristics

Children with fragile X syndrome have a number of positive behavioral characteristics. They are often described as sweet and loving, with a strong desire for social interactions, despite a shy nature. They have a good sense of humor and enjoy jokes and silly games and songs.

Children with fragile X also have a variety of behavioral challenges. Hatton, Hooper, Bailey, Skinner, Sullivan, and Wheeler (2002) found that 49% of boys ages 4-12 scored within the borderline or clinical range on the total problem behavior scale of the *Child Behavior Checklist (CBCL)*

(Achenbach, 1991). It was also found that 56-57% scored in the borderline or clinical range on the attention and thought problem subscales, and 26% scored in those ranges on the social problems subscales. They report that thought problems, social problems, and poor attention appear to contribute to the elevated total problem scores. The items on the thought problem scale particularly tap into the autistic-like behaviors of individuals with fragile X.

Recent research has shown that behavior problems in boys are also connected to their environments, specifically to educational and therapeutic services. Hessl, Dyer-Friedman, Glaser, Wisbeck, Barajas, Taylor, and Reiss (2001) found that mothers who rate educational and therapeutic interventions as effective for their boys with fragile X also report fewer behavioral problems in those children. This area of research is quite new, and clearly new knowledge about the interactions of genetic and environmental factors is of great importance to educators and therapists.

. . . mothers who rate educational and therapeutic interventions as effective for their boys with fragile X also report fewer behavioral problems in those children.

Attention Deficit/Hyperactivity Disorder

Attention deficit/hyperactivity disorder (ADHD) is very common in boys with fragile X. ADHD is a neurologically-based condition that causes difficulties in the ability to focus and maintain attention, control impulsivity, ignore distractions, and control the urge to move about and be physically active. In a review of various research studies, R. Hagerman (2002b) reports that anywhere from 47-100% of boys with fragile X have various features of ADHD. Many boys meet the criteria for the three components of ADHD-C (combined type), as defined in the *Diagnostic and Statistical Manual* (*DSM-IV*) (American Psychiatric Association, 1994). These criteria are inattentive, hyperactive, and impulsive. Following are some behavioral characteristics through the early years that link ADHD with fragile X:

* Boys with fragile X syndrome are often reported as being very active as young children. Along with language delays, hyperactivity is an early telling characteristic when fragile X is suspected.

* Research with infants shows early indications of difficulty in the ability to guide attention. Problems in this area continue throughout childhood (R. Hagerman, 2002b).

* Boys tend to be easily overstimulated and to have short attention spans.

While the hyperactivity may ease with the onset of puberty, attention problems often remain throughout adulthood (Fryns, 1985). Interestingly, the presence of ADHD seems to counteract some of the shyness and social withdrawal for boys, while girls have fewer

ADHD symptoms and more problems with shyness (Sobesky, Porter, Pennington, and Hagerman, 1995).

R. Hagerman (2002b) states that approximately 35% of girls with fragile X have attention and impulsivity issues without hyperactivity problems. They may be diagnosed as ADHD-I, the predominantly inattentive type. Because they may be quieter in the classroom and may not exhibit the hyperactive behavior of some boys, their learning issues and needs may not be noticed as quickly.

Attention deficit disorders may be tied to the sensory overload issues that affect so many children with fragile X. They may become hyperaroused, nervous, and fidgety, resulting in hyperactivity and impulsive outbursts. More symptoms of ADHD may be seen in settings that are visually and auditorally overwhelming.

Anxiety

Hypervigilance has been tied to anxiety issues for both boys and girls with fragile X, and it may be one of the most common underlying emotional features of fragile X. Belser and Sudhalter (2001) believe that a defect in the autonomic nervous system interferes with the ability to regulate arousal. Sensitivity to environmental features (visual, auditory, and tactile surroundings) and changes in routines cause great worry in many children. They worry about upcoming events, including positive activities to which they have looked forward. Social anxiety seems to persist throughout life for many affected persons (Dykens, Hodapp, and Leckman, 1994).

Sensitivity to environmental features (visual, auditory, and tactile surroundings) and changes in routines cause great worry in many children.

Anxiety is seen in the overall shy nature of children with fragile X. Their poor eye contact, tendency to turn away during handshakes, and difficulties in social situations all speak to their shyness. Yet, most children with fragile X do have a strong desire for social interaction and, unless they demonstrate many of the characteristics of autism, relate to people, particularly those with whom they are familiar and comfortable.

Higher functioning and older persons with fragile X may be more aware of their differences from other adolescents and worry about their competence, performance, and acceptability. They have enough cognitive awareness to know that they are different, and their anxiety often comes through in the form of self-deprecating comments.

Behavioral Outbursts

Anxiety may escalate into outbursts or tantrums, particularly with males. An inability to filter sensory information seems to cause a rise in emotions that may result in an emotional display. Periodic aggressive outbursts are seen in up to 75% of adolescent males (Saunders, 2001) and are one of the biggest reasons for placement in special education classes. Anxiety is shown by a number of physical signs, some of which may give parents and educators cues before outbursts take place. Here are some examples of behaviors that are physical signs of anxiety:

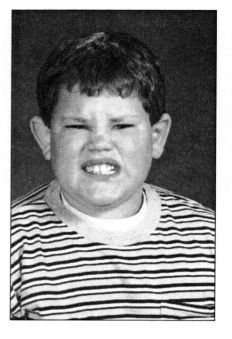

* flapping hands with stress or excitement

* biting hands or clothing

* stiffening the body

* clenching hands

* turning red in the face

* averting eye contact

* beginning long repetitions of perseverative, irrelevant language

* whining, crying, or misbehaving in order to get out of overwhelming situations.

Mood swings and disruptive behavior may take place most often during intense, demanding, or overwhelming experiences, including loud situations, transitions, crowded conditions, or requests for greetings or public speaking. Positive attention may even cause embarrassment and then panic (Braden, 2002c).

Aggressive behaviors or outbursts may involve both avoidance and escape behaviors (Braden, 2002c). During outbursts, boys may hit themselves, other children, or teachers, or boys may lash out at objects around them. Self-injurious behaviors, particularly hand-biting, were reported by 58% of families surveyed by Symons, Clark, Hatton, Skinner, and Bailey (2003). These outbursts do not seem to last into adulthood, but rather, decrease over the adolescent years.

Autism

There are a number of overlapping characteristics between fragile X syndrome and autism. While most persons with fragile X show some autistic-like characteristics, and fall somewhere on the autism spectrum, most do not meet the *DSM-IV* (American Psychiatric Association, 1994) diagnostic criteria for autism. Somewhere between 15-28% of persons with fragile X meet all the diagnostic criteria for autism (R. Hagerman, 2002a). In the 1980s, many researchers thought there was a common genetic root for autism and fragile X, but the multiple genetic and environmental causes of autism continue to be explored. Overlapping characteristics include:

* perseveration in speech and actions
* difficulty with social interactions
* shyness
* poor eye contact
* poor play skills
* repetitive, self-stimulating motor behaviors
* some echolalia
* hand flapping
* hand biting

There are some differences, such as the following, between children diagnosed with autism and the children with fragile X who do not meet the diagnostic criteria for autism:

* *attachment:* Children with fragile X are usually seen as having appropriate attachment to caregivers. They will stay in close proximity to those with whom they are familiar, and they seem to differentiate their gaze aversion, according to familiarity with the person involved in the interaction.

* *resistance to environmental changes:* Children with fragile X usually don't have the resistance to small environmental changes (e.g. moving a piece of furniture) that children with autism may have.

* *emotion recognition:* Children with fragile X are better than their peers with autism at identifying emotions in pictures and faces.

It may be that anxiety and sensory overload cause the "autistic-like" symptoms, rather than autism itself, for those who are not truly autistic. Within the fragile X population, those diagnosed with autism seem to have more severe cognitive and behavioral characteristics.

Emotional Issues in Girls

Girls with fragile X may have specific difficulties in the areas of behavior and emotional development. They are often described as shy, and they may have difficulty with social contacts. Their interpersonal comfort level is negatively affected by excess people, demands, and stimuli. Keysor, Mazzocco, McLeod, and Hoehn-Saric (2002) describe girls with fragile X as having a heightened state of arousal when compared to a control group. In an experimental setting, they had arousal and anxiety symptoms even before being asked to complete arithmetic, attention, and risk-taking tasks.

. . . only a small percentage of persons with fragile X have psychoses, but inappropriate diagnosis may be made if observers confuse psychosis with the self-talk, gesturing, and other odd mannerisms of fragile X.

Some girls with fragile X have schizotypal behaviors, including poor eye contact, odd mannerisms, and hand stereotypies. R. Hagerman (2002a) says that only a small percentage of persons with fragile X have psychoses, but inappropriate diagnosis may be made if observers confuse psychosis with the self-talk, gesturing, and other odd mannerisms of fragile X.

With their diagnosis of nonverbal learning disabilities, many girls may have a variety of social cognition problems. As part of their executive function disorders, they may not judge social situations well and appear socially inappropriate. Depression, paranoia, and problems with mood lability have also been reported in some girls and women with fragile X (Sobesky et al., 1994).

Diagnosis of Emotional and Behavioral Disorders

The diagnosis of emotional and behavioral disorders in children with fragile X must be based upon multiple sources of information: medical, observational, standardized, individually-administered tests, and checklists and rating scales. Optimal intervention involves a combination of special education, various individual and small group types of therapy, and medical monitoring.

Medical Considerations

A medical diagnosis by a physician — perhaps a pediatric neurologist — familiar with the syndrome, is of great importance. Anxiety symptoms, behavioral problems, and ADHD may be very responsive to medication. While there is no cure for fragile X syndrome at this time, medical intervention can provide effective treatment for many of the symptoms. The web address www.fragilex.org/html/medications.htm (R. Hagerman 2002b) reviews a number of medications that have proven to be successful in helping to relieve emotional and behavioral symptoms in children and adults with fragile X. Families, educators, and physicians may need to analyze the effectiveness of a number of medications before finding the proper combinations. Serotonin reuptake inhibitors (SSRIs) and stimulants designed for ADHD have proven successful with many persons with fragile X.

Educational Considerations

Individual behavioral intervention plans must be based upon a careful analysis of a variety of areas and their interactions. In addition to seeking medical input, educators, school social workers, school psychologists, and therapists can complete evaluations of emotional and behavioral development. Adaptive behavior checklists can help pinpoint needs in the areas of daily living skills, socialization, thinking and problem solving, attention, and independence.

There is no one test to diagnose ADHD, but an evaluation of emotional, educational, and social development, in addition to the medical exam, is helpful. Checklists for the characteristics of ADHD are useful in analyzing patterns across a day and in various settings, with particular reference to stressful situations and demands.

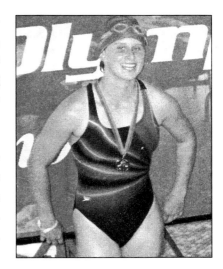

Autism rating scales may also be useful in the determination of most salient autism characteristics. While many children with fragile X do not meet all the criteria for autism, these rating scales may be helpful in developing the most appropriate goals for a number of autistic-like behaviors.

Intervention Techniques

Individual behavioral intervention plans require the combined inputs of parents, teachers, social workers, school psychologists, and therapists in order to design the most effective goals and strategies. These behavioral plans must take into account the variety of factors that specifically affect persons with fragile X syndrome. It is also appropriate to incorporate social skills training, goals regarding sensory and environmental inputs, calming activities, and individual counseling.

Attention Deficit/Hyperactivity Disorder

Treatment of attention deficit/hyperactivity disorders in children with fragile X involves the same strategies used with other children with ADHD, but with special attention to the sensory overload issues experienced by those with fragile X. An evaluation by a pediatric neurologist may result in a medication trial with one of the stimulant medications used for ADHD.

✳ *Environmental Factors*

In addition to medication, evaluation of the environment and triggers for hyperactivity and distractibility may result in specific alterations of the classroom schedule that can make an important difference for those with ADHD. Here are some examples of simple changes that can be made:

- rearranging the order of classes and/or subjects in order to create a balance of active and sedentary activities

- presenting short lessons with adequate breaks

- altering seating placement to reduce distractors

- removing or reducing distractions present in the classroom

✳ *Behavioral Plans*

Behavioral plans with clear behavioral expectations and rewards can be effective for ADHD issues. Token reward systems that incorporate earning stickers or points for acceptable behavior that can be traded for valued activities have proven successful with many children with fragile X (Braden, 2000b). Such behavioral plans must necessarily be written at a level of understanding for each child with fragile X.

✳ *Physical Movement*

Activities that involve physical movement can also be built into the day to alleviate some of the student's restlessness and distractibility:

- sharpening a pencil

- taking trash to the wastebasket

- delivering a message to the office

Additional activities can include heavy work that supports sensory input:

- delivering a case of milk cartons to the kindergarten class

- taking a stack of books to the library

- loading juice bottles into a machine

Physical activities can also be incorporated into language and social skills goals that involve carrying out specific tasks and asking questions or giving information to someone else.

Anxiety

Strategies that help a child with fragile X to feel more knowledgeable and in control of the happenings around him or her will lessen anxiety.

* *Scheduling*
  - A visual schedule (pictures or words), such as a pocket chart, is essential for the classroom and therapy rooms. Changes in the schedule might be signaled with a special colored insert.

  - Provide parents with written schedules of upcoming activities. They need to be kept informed of upcoming changes so that everyone involved can use the same words and information to explain planned assemblies, concerts, field trips, and emergency drills.

  - If participation in crowded or loud events is too overwhelming at first, make backup plans for a child's return to a quieter classroom with an aide. Goals should gradually support the child's ability to take part in crowded or noisy activities.

* *Visual Aids*
  - Use flow charts, lists, and pictures to itemize activities within a lesson so that a child will have a sense of control over the length and type of activities involved.

  - Visual cues are also helpful as signals and may include a covered mouth for "quiet" or simple elements of sign language.

- Visual props can prepare students for activities outside the classroom. For example, have students preview a menu before visiting a restaurant or look through a programs before attending a play or performance. This written information will help a child understand the expectations of an upcoming event.

- Use visual props with a language and social skills role-play to help the child understand each component of the event. You might lead a student through a program for a musical performance and say, "We will listen to the band. They will play these four songs. We will be quiet while they play their songs. After each song, we will clap. When the program is over, we will go back to our classroom."

✱ *Narrowing Choices*

Some children with fragile X seem to become overwhelmed by too many choices, even when the choices are of a positive nature. Anxiety builds up when the child is faced with an over-whelming library of books, a video store full of tapes, a restaurant with too many choices on the menu, or too many fun activities from which to choose. Teachers and parents may need to help the child narrow the field by offering a choice of just two or three items.

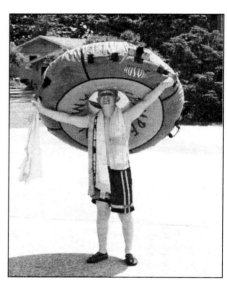

Behavioral Outbursts

There is little research regarding the effectiveness of specific behavioral interventions, so many reports rely on clinical observations. Braden (2000b) and Hills Epstein, Riley, and Sobesky (2002) recommend the ABC approach, an analysis of antecedents, behaviors, and consequences. Braden (2000b) recommends videotaping the child in the classroom or therapy room and then observing the social demands and environmental stimuli that precede an outburst. Reviewing the video for loud noises and voices, changes in routines, difficult academic requirements, or overwhelming social situations may provide clues for preventing behavioral outbursts.

$\mathcal{A}$ntecedents
$\mathcal{B}$ehavior
$\mathcal{C}$onsequences

Awareness of the antecedents to a crisis, including the physical symptoms shown by children who are becoming agitated, can often prevent a behavioral outburst. Children may stiffen up; tighten their hands; become red in the face; flap their arms; begin long, rapid bursts of speech; or pull their shirts over their heads. Intervention for preventing outbursts might include the following:

* removal of the child from overwhelming situations

* reduction of overwhelming inputs

* use of soft voices and calming language

* provision of calming spaces, including bean bag chairs, small forts, or carrels equipped with music CDs or books on tape

* provision of tactile inputs: deep pressure on shoulders, papoose wrap in a blanket, big ball to bounce on, tubing or candy for chewing

* work with anxiety reduction strategies: deep breathing, muscle relaxation

* introduction of a distraction: song, counting, familiar story

Social Skills

Pragmatic, or conversational disorders are common to both boys and girls with fragile X syndrome. Shyness, anxiety, attention deficit disorders, and sensory overload all contribute to pragmatic disorders. Thus, social skills training is a vital piece of the IEP for most children with fragile X. Social skills goals may be designed jointly by social workers, special educators, occupational therapists, and speech-language pathologists.

The importance of social skills cannot be overstated, as they are related to so many aspects of life (Szymanski, 2003):

* personal development and identity

* employability, productivity, and career success

* quality of life, physical health, psychological health, and the ability to cope with stress

Without direct instruction, children with fragile X syndrome may not develop their maximum levels of social competence. While some may never be comfortable in many social interactions, they can make progress in a variety of skills.

✳ *Published Programs*

A number of social skills programs target conversational skills and other interactive behaviors. With these materials, children must understand what skill is being targeted and then work through observations, role-plays, guided conversations, and clearly-defined tasks.

✳ *Adult Interactions*

As social skills goals necessitate interactions among people, various adults can be briefed and targeted to work with students on particular skills:

• The secretary in the school office can look for eye contact and a greeting when the student with fragile X delivers the daily attendance report.

• School maintenance personnel can expect a greeting and relevant question about the day's job when students are assigned a work task with them.

✳ *Peer Group Interactions*

Social interaction groups with children may need to start with behavioral and social expectations for appropriate group behavior. These basic interaction behaviors, such as maintaining eye contact and turn-taking, may be ones that other children learn intuitively or through observation, but that children with fragile X and autism-spectrum disorders do not. Group behaviors should be taught in a calm, verbal, and direct manner, with visual cues for turn-taking (such as a talking stick) or quiet mouth (such as a hand over mouth signal). New situations in groups can be previewed and rehearsed with structured practice and scripts (see Chapter 4: Speech and Language).

✳ *Social Stories*

Social stories (Gray, 1995) have proven to be successful with a variety of goals for children with fragile X. Social stories may be used to help a child process a situation and implement a solution. They are usually short stories written with descriptive sentences, reaction sentences, and solution sentences. They may describe a particular situation in which the child has some difficulty and offers positive solutions (often, an "I will try . . ." statement).

Gagnon's (2001) *Power Cards* use some of the same principles, but also engage the child's interest by having a favorite person, character, or star as the motivator. In short stories and summaries on a card, the Brady Bunch, Power Rangers, or Barbie might tell the child how important it is to accomplish a certain task.

Conclusions

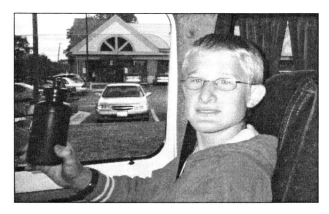

Behavioral problems are common in children with fragile X syndrome and are often of more concern to educators and parents than any other area of functioning. In order to develop effective intervention approaches, behavioral problems must be seen in the context of all areas of development: cognitive, sensory, and language. For children who have difficulty expressing themselves, who are overwhelmed by a variety of sensory experiences throughout the day, and who are not able to comprehend many situations, directions, and emotions around them, emotional responses and inappropriate behaviors may be understandable. For the adults who live and work with them, seeing the behaviors as part of a larger picture will help with appropriate, sensitive, and effective strategies.

chapter 7 *Educational Programming*

Finding effective educational and therapeutic personnel and appropriate settings for all children with special needs is critical. For children with fragile X syndrome, there are several important considerations that need to be taken into account. Most boys and many girls with fragile X require special education and therapeutic services throughout their childhood years, and the choices of teachers, therapists, and settings may have great impact on their development.

Early Intervention

Many children with fragile X enter early intervention (birth to three) programs due to delays in speech and language development or motor skills. Many parents do not know that their child has fragile X syndrome when the child enters the birth to three programs, but they do recognize delays in development. Bailey, Skinner and Sparkman (2003) found in a survey of 274 families that many parents became concerned about developmental delays when their children were about 13 months old. However, a professional confirmation of that concern did not take place until the children were 21 months old, and a fragile X diagnosis was not made until around 32 months. Thus, valuable time in early intervention may have been lost, as 25% of the parents were being told to "wait and see" because their child's development might improve without intervention.

Many parents do not know that their child has fragile X syndrome when the child enters the birth to three programs, but they do recognize delays in development.

Early intervention was added to federal law in 1986 to encourage states to set up programs for infants and toddlers and their families. The Secretary of Education makes grants to states to implement and maintain statewide services through Part C, the Early Intervention for Infants and Toddlers with Disabilities and Their Families Amendment to the Individuals with Disabilities Education Act (IDEA). The goals of Part C are to meet the individual needs of children and families, to enhance the development of young children, and to minimize the need for special education through early intervention. Children qualify for such early intervention if they have developmental delays, physical or mental conditions with a high probability of resulting in developmental delays, or at-risk factors.

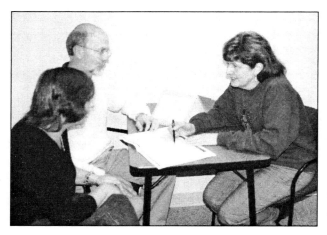

Unlike special education services from ages 3-21, early intervention is not the responsibility of the local public schools. Parents are referred to a variety of local providers in their area, often coordinated by "child find" or "child and family connections" personnel. Early intervention services may be provided in homes, centers, or hospitals. Goals are very family centered, with parent education a major part of the therapies. Parents and caregivers are supported in encouraging their child to learn and grow, assisted in obtaining services, counseled in areas of need, and helped with the transition to early childhood (ages 3-5) programs. Services might include vision and hearing testing, occupational therapy, physical therapy, speech and language services, audiology services, social work and psychological services, nutrition counseling, medical evaluations, and assistive technology (Anderson, Chitwood, and Hayden, 1997).

An Individualized Family Service Plan (IFSP) is developed for each child and family, with reviews every six months. Each state has its own format for the IFSP and its own eligibility requirements for qualifying for early intervention. Eligibility often consists of a significant delay in development in one or more areas.

Most boys with fragile X syndrome show developmental delays in their first or second year of life. If their parents know about early intervention services, they can access the help of early intervention providers. Therapists can then help them provide early stimulation in effective ways for cognitive, sensory, speech and language, and behavioral development. Siblings of diagnosed children may also be at risk for fragile X and thus may be eligible from birth for early intervention services.

For children with fragile X syndrome, therapies and parent education should focus on the assessments and interventions that are most appropriate for the individual child with this syndrome. Assessments are not necessarily formal, standardized tests, but rather, may be rating scales, structured observations, parent and caregiver reports, and medical histories. Physical and occupational therapists may assess sensory and motor planning issues, while speech-language pathologists determine if there is a need to add sign language or augmentative communication to the interaction of adults and an infant or toddler with fragile X. Parents may be taught techniques for calming, strategies for establishing routines, ideas for the stimulation of communication, and cognitive development activities. Even at this very young age, it is important to introduce visual cues and predictable routines. From the beginning, the integration of services, such as occupational and speech and language therapy, provides the optimal stimulation.

The speech-language pathologist and occupational therapist can help parents work with their child's sucking and eating skills. Oral motor work may begin early to develop the abilities to suck, chew, and swallow. The early interventionist and speech-language pathologist also go into the home or center to help the infant or toddler develop communication skills and to help the parents develop communication systems with their children (Moore-Brown and Montgomery, 2001).

Parents may need to be taught interactive games, such as "Peek-a-boo" and "Pat-a-cake," if they are not already doing these activities with their children. The SLP and OT may also work with parents on joint attention, infant's or toddler's communication functions, and pre-verbal requests, rejections, and comments. Braden (2000a) suggests that attention is an important area for young children with fragile X, but that attending behaviors should be encouraged rather than forced, due to the anxiety issues of many of these children. She suggests developing attention through turn-taking, game playing, music, and finger plays. Parallel talk techniques can be used to help parents comment on what they or the child is doing while playing, thus encouraging language stimulation rather than demands for language output.

The first transition that takes place for a child and family involved in birth to three programs is the move from early intervention to early childhood education when the child turns three.

The first transition that takes place for a child and family involved in birth to three programs is that of the move from early intervention to early childhood education following the child's third birthday. This is a major transition for both the child and the family, as many children with special education needs begin their first school experience at age three. The early intervention (EI) team may update assessments or work with the early childhood education (ECE) team to provide a new evaluation. Early intervention providers can help parents with the transition by discussing future placement options with them and encouraging them to visit local early childhood programs. The child can continue to have an IFSP or begin with an Individual Educational Plan (IEP) once he or she enters ECE.

Early Childhood Education

Once the child turns three, services are mandated through the public school system for those who qualify. These services are often provided, with transportation, in local public schools. As a result, the child and family are often facing many new routines. Early childhood education may be provided in classrooms that serve children with a variety of special needs, or it may be provided in nursery schools or daycares with special education supports from the local public schools. As long as the child with fragile X has some children around him or her to serve as models (children with more expressive language or calm behaviors), either type of setting can be very effective. In either of these settings, an IFSP or IEP with "functional outcomes" must be in place to govern the child's goals and intervention.

A number of factors make early childhood education most successful and appropriate for the child with fragile X. The structure of the classroom, style of the staff, ability of classmates to serve as models, and the curriculum are all important to the early childhood setting that is chosen.

Classroom Structure and Scheduling

Staff members need to be aware of both classroom structure and levels of stimulation. Children with fragile X and autism thrive on structure and routine and do less well with visually or auditorally overwhelming classrooms and activities. For example, walls that are completely covered in stimulating decorations may be visually overwhelming for such children. Likewise, crowded or messy activity centers, tables, and desks may prove to be disturbing. Saunders (2001) recommends structuring the environment with calm spaces and calm, quiet voices. Visual cues and schedules (with both pictures and words) can create a sense of order and routine for children with sensory overload and attention deficit-hyperactivity disorder issues.

Children with fragile X and autism thrive on structure and routine and do less well with visually or auditorally overwhelming classrooms and activities.

Scheduling that takes into account the attention deficit-hyperactivity disorders of children with fragile X can make for a more effective day. Short activities that alternate between sitting and movement may be helpful. Allowing children to move about regularly can prevent some behavioral outbursts and tantrums. As part of the overall routine, many early childhood classes have "jobs" for each student. For the student with fragile X, these might include movement activities, such as collecting the markers after an activity and putting them on the shelves, carrying the wastebasket around after a snack to collect napkins and cups, or cleaning up a center after free play time.

Curriculum

Classroom based and collaborative consultation models with integrated curriculum and service delivery are often most effective for children with fragile X. Early childhood teachers, speech-language pathologists, occupational therapists, physical therapists, and parents can all design an integrated curriculum. Speech-language pathologists and occupational therapists need to be aware of early childhood development and curriculum, while early childhood teachers should have knowledge of normal speech-language and motor development.

Ongoing collaboration can result in activities that address a number of goals: attention and behavior, speech-language, motor, and pre-academic. The curriculum can build on the strengths of children with fragile X:

- good receptive vocabularies
- good visual memories
- strong imitation skills
- sense of humor
- relatively good gross motor skills.

At the same time, their weaknesses can be addressed:

- attention deficit-hyperactivity disorder
- impulsivity
- organizational skills
- expressive language
- pragmatics
- sequential memory
- counting and math concepts
- abstract reasoning

Activities can be designed that address weaknesses while utilizing strengths. For instance, story time, with books such as *Rosie's Walk* by Pat Hutchins, can include work on language comprehension of prepositions (as Rosie goes *over*, *around*, and *under* various objects), motor skills (as children act out Rosie's walk), and sequencing (as children follow her route). Books such as *The Very Hungry Caterpillar* by Eric Carle can be used to focus on numbers (as the caterpillar eats one more item each day) and days of the week. The physical or occupational therapist designs the motor sequence of activities, while the early childhood special educator and speech-language pathologist work on the language comprehension and expression goals. Print-related activities (e.g., use of big books) can be used to encourage pre-reading skills.

Occupational therapy goals that focus on posture, body awareness, balance, and coordination can be pursued with many children, not just those with fragile X. Occupational therapists may train other team members about ways to reduce sensory defensiveness, and to improve sensory awareness, attention, and concentration (Saunders, 2001). Occupational therapists may also provide fine motor activities for the entire class.

Curriculum that taps into IEP goals for social skills may make team members aware of creating opportunities for social interactions. For instance, at snack time, a child with fragile X might be asked to pass out the napkins while establishing brief eye contact with each child and saying, signing, or activating an augmentative device to give a routine greeting (e.g., "One for you"). One-to-one correspondence is developed as a pre-math skill, and both language and fine motor skills are targeted.

Role of Parents

While parents may not have the same direct involvement in their child's activities once the child moves from early intervention to early childhood, they still need to be kept involved as team members. Some early childhood programs use a four-day week for the children, with Fridays reserved for rotating home visits. Such visits allow time for parents and staff members to share updates and reflections on progress and challenges.

On a weekly or monthly basis, parents can be sent schedules of the thematic units, classroom goals, planned field trips, and other important news. Not only can they reinforce themes and goals with the books and games they choose at home, they can also be aware of changes in routine that affect their child's moods. On a daily basis, parents and staff members should send a notebook back and forth from home to school, with a simple checklist or comment about the child's day. The notebook can be as simple as a set of facial expressions regarding various aspects of the day (e.g., smiling face for good behavior) or as thorough as a paragraph or two about an accomplishment of the day. Parents can send back a brief note or picture of an activity at home or any unusual events that may affect the child's school day.

Elementary School

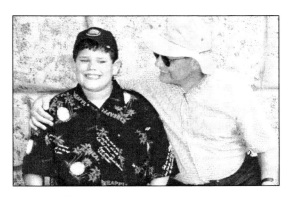

The next major transition for children in special education and their families occurs when children move from early childhood education to a kindergarten or elementary school program. For both families and children, this is another major change: schedules move to full day, settings may change, parents are even less physically present in classrooms, and home visits are unusual. A number of choices must be made about the appropriate education in the least restrictive environment for each child with special needs.

For children with fragile X, the most appropriate settings for elementary education may vary widely. Schools are to provide a continuum of services, and parents and staff need to match the child's needs with services on that continuum. Needs may change over the child's school years, and the setting that is chosen for early childhood or primary school may not be appropriate for junior high or high school. The balance of an academic focus and functional/life skills goals needs to be examined with each annual revision of the IEP, and it is the IEP that should govern the services and setting.

Staff and Classroom Characteristics

There are some very important considerations to keep in mind when choosing the most appropriate placement for a child with fragile X. Saunders (2001) refers to the areas that are most important for the staff of the classroom: people who understand fragile X syndrome and the particular needs of the individual child because of it; staff who are calm and structured; sufficient staff for support of the child; and staff with knowledge and expertise to plan and implement programs of learning appropriate to the developmental level of the child. Symons, Clark, and Roberts (2001) found that the classroom engagement of elementary school children with fragile X syndrome was strongly related to the environmental and instructional quality of the teachers and classrooms. The ways in which the

The ways in which the teachers structured and arranged the classroom environment was much more important to student engagement than were specific aspects of the child's fragile X status

teachers structured and arranged the classroom environment was much more important to student engagement than were specific aspects of the child's fragile X status (such as severity, medication usage, and dual diagnosis with autism).

Other important classroom components to consider include spatial, auditory, and visual aspects:

* *Spatially*, the room should not be crowded, and there need to be some quiet, nondistracting places for the child to work.

* *Auditorally*, the most appropriate classroom is quiet and soothing.

* *Visually*, the classroom should not be overloaded with decorations, but daily schedules can be posted and referred to often.

Settings

The choice of most appropriate educational settings depends upon the individual characteristics and needs of each child. Because boys and girls with fragile X may vary in their levels of severity, appropriate placements for them may differ. For girls who are minimally affected by fragile X, an inclusive setting or regular education class with a resource room and special education services on a regular basis may be most effective. For other girls with more severe involvement, a special education room, coupled with some mainstream classes, may be less anxiety provoking and more appropriate.

Boys with fragile X vary widely in their educational needs. Some might be educated in regular education classes, with adequate supports, while others are more appropriately educated in self-contained special education placements, which serve children at a particular level of functioning. In regular education rooms, boys will likely need the services of speech-language pathologists, occupational therapists, special educators, and teaching assistants. It may be the role of these persons to decide what parts of the curriculum are appropriate and to adapt that curriculum for the child with fragile X. Services may be offered in combinations of classroom-based and/or small group intervention (e.g., the SLP works on pre-teaching vocabulary to a group of children before a unit on social studies; the OT provides some calming activities before a quiet listening task) or pull-out approaches.

Inclusive regular education classrooms provide an opportunity to make classmates aware of how to be friends with the child who has fragile X. Some younger elementary school children may believe that they can "catch fragile X" and need some basic information about the causes of their classmate's learning differences. Children's books, such as *My Brother Has Fragile X* (Steiger, 1998) can be used to help discussion about the affected child, and programs such as Circle of Friends (Snow and Hasbury, 1989) provide classmates with ways in which to be friends.

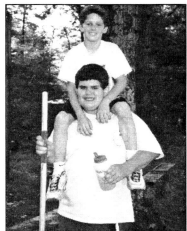

Special education classrooms may be designed for children with various levels of functioning. Goals may be centered around academics or around functional living activities. In either setting, practical, functional goals, such as math activities regarding the use of money, ability to tell time, and accuracy in measurement, should be included.

Junior High and High School Services

The transitions to junior high or middle school and then to high school are often major ones. The schools may be much larger; in special education settings, changing classes may even be required. New students come to the school from a variety of "feeder" schools, and setting, teachers, and students are all unfamiliar once again. For students who qualify for extended year services, summer school may be a good time to become acclimated to the new setting. Otherwise, an orientation and tour before school begins may be very welcome to both the student with fragile X and his or her parents. Braden (2000a) recommends such a visit to help reduce anxiety and to give the student a clearer visual picture of the new setting and expectations. The family might take photographs and create a book that illustrates the new people, classrooms, and other school locales the student will encounter. Once the school schedule is formulated, the parents can find pictures that match daily activities and "walk" the adolescent through the daily schedule.

Transitional Plans

By the time a student in special education reaches age 14, transitional plans for adulthood are often begun; by age 16, these plans need to be in place. IDEA requires a "coordinated set of activities for a student, designed with an outcome-oriented process that promotes movement from school to post-school activities" (Pierangelo and Crane, 1997, p. 4). Forming long-range goals and designing junior high and high school experiences that meet those goals are all part of transition services and become the basis of the Individualized Transitional Education Program (ITEP). Many decisions regarding combinations of academic and vocational courses, special education and inclusion courses, and daily living goals must be made and put into place. These decisions need to be made with the involvement of the adolescent who has special needs.

It is at the middle school or junior high level that many families of adolescents with fragile X decide that more intensive special education services must be in place.

It is at the middle school or junior high level that many families of adolescents with fragile X decide that more intensive special education services (which focus on pre-vocational and vocational skills, language and social skills, and practical, functional math skills) must be in place. Some boys who have been in regular education, inclusionary settings, may move into special education programs focused on their particular needs and outcomes. In such special education settings, the focus may be on the following:

* community access

* living options

* leisure skills

* vocational placements

* functional academic goals (Braden, 2000a)

Girls with fragile X may be able to remain in regular education classes with resource assistance in their more challenging subjects. They and their families may also choose to move toward special education placements that provide more support in non-academic areas. These girls and their parents also have decisions to make about community and four-year colleges, vocational choices and training, living options, leisure skills, and community involvement.

Vocational Assessments and Placements

One of the major areas for high school special education to address is that of vocational assessments and placements. Even in junior high or middle school, young teens may begin a variety of pre-vocational work experiences to see what jobs they prefer and which ones they do well. Staff use what they know about a young teen's verbal reasoning, reading levels, writing abilities, spatial discrimination, social skills, interests, and attention to determine good matches to specific jobs. Some students with fragile X prefer jobs without a good deal of language interaction (e.g., collating and stapling papers in the office, putting juice cans in the machine). For others, the pre-vocational activities can include language goals (e.g., delivering handouts or picking up attendance sheets, and greeting the teachers).

By high school, a more formal vocational assessment must take place. Pierangelo and Crane (1997) recommend a three-level vocational assessment:

1. Collecting information about the adolescent (such as achievements and interests)

2. Assessing aptitudes, strengths, and weaknesses

3. Evaluating the adolescent in real or simulated job experiences

Work and training options might include unpaid internships and apprenticeships, as well as "real world" placements in the local community. Job coaches, who may be special education teachers, vocational education teachers, or speech-language pathologists, accompany students to employment settings to help with expectations of the job and to foster skills for success in that position.

The special education team, including the parents and the adolescent with fragile X, must ultimately decide whether the long-range goal is for competitive employment, supported employment (which might include a job coach), or sheltered employment (usually in non-profit agencies, with all workers having disabilities). For some higher functioning adolescents with fragile X, post-secondary education might include vocational centers, trade and technical schools, and community colleges. For others, the transition to the world of work will take place at age 21, when secondary schooling is no longer an option.

For some higher functioning adolescents with fragile X, post-secondary education might include vocational centers, trade and technical schools, and community colleges.

Related Services

Adolescents with fragile X syndrome may still qualify for a variety of related services during junior high and high school, including speech/language services, occupational therapy, and behavior intervention. The speech-language pathologist coordinates a variety of academic and life skills activities for junior high and high school students with fragile X syndrome. Some junior high and high schools offer social skills classes as credit bearing courses. In these classes, skills such as making phone calls, interviewing for jobs, asking a friend to a movie, or asking a teacher or employer a question, can be emphasized. Other schools offer language arts classes for groups of high school students with special needs in which SLPs conduct class periods regarding vocabulary, reading and writing, and the language of math. Pull-out therapy for specific speech and language skills may no longer be appropriate or helpful for generalization of those skills outside the therapy room.

Sensory and behavioral goals can also be addressed in classroom-based and consultative ways. Occupational therapists and behavior disorder specialists serve as consultants to and team partners with others working on calming techniques. They may have roles in the vocational choices recommended as they assess and work with issues of sensory overload. Behavioral intervention plans, with attention to scheduling, vocational and academic activities, and staff and classroom styles, can be best designed by all team members working with the adolescent with fragile X.

Conclusions

With attention to effective teaching and appropriate settings, children and adolescents with fragile X can make tremendous progress. Knowledge of the etiology of fragile X syndrome and the characteristics that result from it are helpful to staff and parents in planning effective academic intervention for each child.

chapter 8

Academic Intervention

In this book, we have previously addressed cognitive development, sensory processing, speech and language, and behaviors in children with fragile X syndrome. Each of these areas requires attention and impacts the others. There are also academic areas that require special knowledge for most effectively teaching the child or adolescent with fragile X syndrome. While there is a wide range of functioning among these children, there are similarities in their learning and processing styles that require specific teaching strategies.

Teaching to Cognitive Strengths

Braden (2000a, 2000b), Mirrett, Roberts, and Price (2003) and Saunders (2001) all speak to building on the cognitive strengths of children with fragile X while also addressing instruction to their cognitive weaknesses. Building on cognitive strengths involves some attention to the modality and manner of presentation and may be the reason why achievement is often higher than aptitude scores for children with fragile X.

Building on cognitive strengths involves some attention to the modality and manner of presentation and may be the reason why achievement is often higher than aptitude scores for children with fragile X.

From a survey of speech-language pathologists who work with young boys having fragile X, Mirrett et al. (2003) report that teaching through visual modeling and imitation, with frequent visual prompts, such as pictures, drawings, and simple signs, is most effective. Modeling an activity, supplementing auditory directions with objects and pictures, using real objects and videos, and adding a simple visual sign to a series of directions can all ensure success with a lesson.

Both Braden (2002a) and Saunders (2001) recommend using tasks that focus on simultaneous processing, such as whole words and completed objects, before attempting to break tasks into sequential steps. A simultaneous style of teaching may run counter to a teacher's usual practice; rather than teaching individual steps and putting them together later, children with fragile X often need to be taught the entire process first, with repetition of the whole. For instance, a teacher might present a science activity as a completed project and then broken down into parts. When teaching children to write their names, the instructor can present the entire name in a dot-to-dot format, even if the student is only required to write the first letter and trace the others.

Saunders recommends teaching through practical experiences. In a survey of special education teachers (1999), she found that the children with fragile X had a preference for practical work, especially activities that involve physical effort. They preferred and were most successful with activities that met these criteria:

* short length of time
* do not involve lengthy sitting and listening
* limited need for direct verbal communication

Saunders (1999) and Mirrett, et al. (2003) suggest activities that focus on high interest areas and involve concrete, hands-on experiences, active experimentation, multimodality presentations, physical manipulation, and acting.

Teaching to Cognitive Weaknesses

Teaching with attention to cognitive and processing weaknesses involves goals addressing these areas:

* *Attention:* Turn-taking, waiting
* *Sequencing:* Following directions in order, putting pictures in order, following steps in math problems, sequencing letters for spelling words, scanning words in reading
* *Memory:* Short-term memory
* *Motor planning and handwriting*
* *Generalization*
* *Self-organization, self-awareness*
* *Slowed processing time* (Braden, 2000a; Saunders, 2001)

To address these weaknesses, Saunders (2001) recommends these general strategies:

- ✳ preparing the child for work
- ✳ non-distracting spaces
- ✳ daily schedules and routines
- ✳ clear, uncluttered worksheets
- ✳ calming strategies

She also recommends using unambiguous tasks with clear beginnings and ends (e.g., if 10 words are to be written, provide a worksheet with 10 numbered spaces). Verbal instructions should be clear, simple, and short, with visual cues (photos, then drawings, and finally, words) when possible. Verbal directions need to increase from one to two and so on, always monitoring for frustrations and successes.

Once information has been made meaningful and stored in long-term memory, it is usually well retrieved by children with fragile X.

Memory strategies might include music, rhythmic repetitions, and visual and color-coded cues for important information, such as phone numbers and addresses. Once information has been made meaningful and stored in long-term memory, it is usually well retrieved by children with fragile X.

Motor planning strategies might target handwriting but also allow for outputs by which a child can show knowledge without having to write. Here are some ways to bypass the difficulty of writing without sacrificing the need for the child to be able to show his or her knowledge:

- ✳ worksheets with simple motor response tasks (e.g., circling, choosing from multiple choices)
- ✳ talking into a tape recorder
- ✳ answering verbally
- ✳ drawing a picture
- ✳ making a chart
- ✳ entering information on a keyboard

Learned tasks should be carried out with various people, in different settings, and with new issues to encourage generalization of information. Braden (2000a) recommends specific work on problem solving with new issues by applying information from previously learned applications.

Self-organization and self-awareness involve levels of metacognitive awareness that may be difficult for some children with fragile X. They need visual cues for organization of activities and sequences. Self-awareness, especially regarding a child's own feelings of stress, can be helped by programs such as, *How Does Your Engine Run?* (Williams and Shellenberger, 1996), which target self-awareness of feelings of stress.

Question–Answer–Question Strategy

Instructor: Where is the refrigerator in your home? Is it in the bathroom or the kitchen?

Pause

The refrigerator is in the kitchen. Where is the refrigerator?

Pause

Student: In the kitchen.

For slow processing time, Saunders (2001) recommends adequate wait time and avoidance of direct questions. Questions with cues, such as multiple-choice options, may be more productive. A "question-answer-question" format may strengthen the processing loop, as the teacher or therapist asks a question, pauses, answers it herself, and repeats it, pausing again for the response.

These strategies for teaching to cognitive strengths and weaknesses of children with fragile X, with attention to processing styles, sensory issues, and speech and language development, are helpful across a variety of academic areas. Effective strategies to guide the teaching of reading, written language, mathematics, other academic areas, and computer literacy are based on all of these areas.

Reading

Many girls with fragile X learn to decode very well and may have good comprehension skills. Some may do much better with literal, rather than inferential, comprehension, but for many, reading is an area of strength. Boys with fragile X have a wide range of reading abilities, with some being classified as non-readers; many being able to read words, phrases, and short passages; and still others attaining the literacy levels needed for reading chapter books, magazines, and newspapers.

Whole Word Approaches

In teaching to strengths, visual, whole word approaches are often recommended for children with fragile X. There have been more "clinical impressions" of the effectiveness of these strategies than research data. Recently, however, Johnson-Glenburg (2003) compared boys with fragile X matched by decoding level to typically developing boys. She found major deficits in the abilities of boys with fragile X to attack nonwords. She hypothesizes that phonological skills, particularly phonemic awareness, are weak in the fragile X population, and these poor skills may affect sequential recall.

Many auditory areas are difficult for pre-readers and readers with fragile X. The abilities to hear differences among sounds, to sound out words, to blend them together, to syllabicate, and to rhyme may all be areas of weakness. If the child cannot break words apart into sounds or blend those sounds into whole words, it will be very difficult for him or her to learn to read by a phonics method. The child might recognize a whole word, such as *cat* and relate it to the animal, but not be able to relate the letters in the word to their component sounds.

A high interest, whole word approach is often most effective. Initially, teach words that are in the child's receptive vocabulary, and choose words that both look and sound very different. Print words in manuscript in clear, well-formed letters. Have children see, hear, and say the words aloud for multisensory reinforcement.

Object-word associations can take place with various items in the room labeled: e.g., *book*, *chair*, *window*. Match pictured and labeled items to to words, and point out labels on boxes and cartons. Braden (1989) recommends using familiar logos, such as those for fast food restaurants. She expands those to simple word families and then to short sentence strips.

In discussing a visual approach to reading, Johnson and Myklebust (1967) also recommend developing short phrases and sentences, such as *big ball, little ball, blue ball*. They then expand the phrases to simple commands written on cards for, "Read and do" activities (e.g., classroom jobs), and then to experience stories, which reflect the happenings of the classroom and may be supplemented with pictures for cues. Such activities can provide simple comprehension tasks as children talk about their activities and plans. Visual materials for reading should be clear, well-spaced, and uncrowded.

Visual materials for reading should be clear, well-spaced, and uncrowded.

Reading Comprehension

The cognitive level of the individual child will guide the goals for reading. Functional reading for some levels of independence may be targeted for children and adolescents who are at beginning levels of reading. These individuals may eventually shop and cook for themselves if they are able to read labels, cooking directions, and grocery lists. The abilities to read and interpret schedules and timetables may help them take public transportation on their own and to read a TV program listing. They may also be able to read captions under pictures in order to enjoy magazines and newspapers.

Children and adolescents with higher reading levels need to focus on some word attack skills, which can aid comprehension. If individual sounds remain difficult for children to discriminate, the level of the meaningful morpheme may be a possible target. Separating a word into syllables and adding meaningful prefixes and/or suffixes can expand the reading vocabulary greatly as illustrated in the box on the right. Johnson and Myklebust (1967) recommend that additional lines between syllables not be used, as they distort the image of the word and may be confusing. A space between word parts can help the child's visual focus and ability to scan those parts.

> ### *Word Attack Skills*
> *Syllable Separation, Prefixes, & Suffixes*
>
> ✳ Begin with a root word:
> **farm**
> Expand the root word with suffixes:
> **farming**　　**farmer**　　**farms**
>
> ✳ Separation of syllables can help both meaningful reading and spelling of multisyllabic words
> **farm**
> **farm　er**
> **farm　ing**

Some boys with fragile X may be hyperlexic, with a much higher ability to recognize words than to comprehend them (Harris-Schmidt and Fast, 1998). Literal comprehension can be targeted, with basic *wh-* questions about passages, and some ability to make inferences may be developed, even if it is never a strength ("What do you think will happen next?" "How is the boy feeling now?"). Reading comprehension activities might be alternated between those that allow the child to look back at the passage (teaching to the strength) and those that require the child to remember and answer a question, without using the passage (teaching to the weakness).

Written outputs, such as answers to reading questions, should be kept simple, in order to be sure that written language difficulties are not interfering with the ability to answer reading comprehension questions. Reading comprehension might be shown by filling in a blank, circling a correct answer, or stating the answer aloud. Activities that combine reading and writing need to be examined in order to determine if successes and failures are based upon the reading requirements or those of written language.

Written Language

Written language is the highest level of language and the last to be learned (Johnson and Myklebust, 1967). Written language requires cognitive development sufficient to understand the written task, some intact levels of receptive language, reading ability, fine motor skills, visual memory for spelling, and sequencing of letters, words, and ideas. Children with fragile X syndrome, particularly boys, may have difficulties with any or all of these areas.

Written language requires direct instruction. Most people do not learn to write without being taught. For children with fragile X, receptive language and reading skills need to be targeted before and during written language lessons.

Written language may be very limited for some boys with moderate or severe cognitive deficits. For them, it may be most productive to limit the amount of writing that is required when the focus is on other areas of learning. Allowing them to circle an answer, draw a picture, answer verbally, or write one word may be the best way by which to assess their language or reading comprehension. It may be important to have them learn to write their signature and other information important for them (e.g., address, parents' names). For other children with fragile X, a variety of written language areas can be addressed.

Visual-Motor Disorders and Writing

For some children with fragile X, there are problems with the visual motor task of writing. Some even have difficulty copying and are described as having *dysgraphia*. Similar to dyspraxia for speech, those with dysgraphia have difficulty with the motor planning and execution of writing and drawing tasks (Johnson and Myklebust, 1967). Both occupational therapists and special education teachers need to observe and then work with posture, pencil grip, and position of paper. Children with such visual motor problems may need kinesthetic strategies, tracing letters in sand and having teachers use hand over hand techniques. They often work best with stencils, templates, tracing activities, dot-to-dots, and simple mazes. Computer keyboarding skills may help them with clarity, spacing, and corrections. For some, limiting the amount of writing demanded eases frustration, and there may be alternate ways by which to judge understanding of academic tasks.

Computer keyboarding skills may help [some students with fragile X] with clarity, spacing, and corrections.

Formulation and Syntax

Most girls and some boys are able to write sentences, paragraphs, and longer passages. Goals may be centered around sentence formulation, beginning with simple sentences, in which the child must only fill in a blank. Gradually, the child can be given only a sentence starter and be expected to complete the remainder of the sentence. Working up to paragraphs may require much guidance, as the child is given a topic sentence, three sentence starters for supporting details, and a closing sentence. Very concrete topics, with much oral discussion beforehand, can be used at first. Here is an example of a simple paragraph format:

"There are three reasons why fall is my favorite season. The first one is _____. The second one is _____. The last one is _____. That is why I like fall."

As visual cues are gradually reduced, more output is expected. Increased output can be targeted at the sentence level or the paragraph level. Some children may be able to monitor sentences and paragraphs for syntactic or formulation errors, but for others, the metalinguistic ability needed for such tasks may be too demanding.

Spelling

Spelling is often an area of relative strength for both girls and boys with fragile X. Because of their strong visual memories for whole words, memorizing spelling words and reproducing them on a computer or handwritten spelling tests may be areas of success. Some children are able to use the spelling list required of the mainstream class, with perhaps fewer words, while others require a list at their reading level. Spelling can then be integrated with reading goals and meanings addressed.

Several visual strategies can help with spelling and focus on the strengths of children with fragile X, while remediating some of the weaknesses with sequencing. Fill-in-the-blank activities can help strengthen visual memory, as children are given partial visual cues. For example, to help children notice

---

Visual Spelling Strategies

✳ *Fill-in-the blank patterning:*

s w i n g s e t

s w ___ ___ ___ s e ___

s ___ ___ ___ ___ s ___ ___

✳ *Syllable/morpheme recognition:*

re ___ a _____   (*recreation*)

add ____   (*addition*)

____ ina _____   (*examination*)

syllables, letter sequences, and number of letters, a pattern may be developed, such as the one shown in the box on the previous page.

With slow dictation, older and higher functioning children and adolescents may be able to recognize syllables or meaningful morphemes to complete words as shown by the second example in the box.

Another strategy using syllables is to write spelling words on cards, then cut them apart at syllable divisions. The child looks for word parts as the scrambled words are set in front of him, but not individual sounds. Again, the teacher or speech-language pathologist can dictate the word slowly and exaggerate the syllables as the child searches for the word parts that go together.

Mathematics

The area of mathematics is often one of difficulty for both boys and girls with fragile X syndrome. As Mazzacco (2001) and Mazzacco and Lachiewicz (2003) state, mathematics performance and achievement are made up of many areas, including the following:

* math concepts and procedures
* language concepts
* spatial knowledge
* processing speed
* memory
* problem solving

Individual Planning

Because success in mathematics depends on the integration of several subskills, it is imperative to know the reasons behind each individual child's problems with math and to design intervention appropriately.

Math is the academic area that poses the most difficulties for many girls. Their nonverbal learning disabilities are displayed in difficulties with time, size, space, order, and distance. Problems in abstraction or higher level thinking skills may also cause difficulties with problem solving, reasoning, estimation, and other conceptual skills. For boys, math is also an area of great difficulty, often in keeping with their cognitive levels, but exacerbated by comprehension problems, visual spatial confusions, and fine motor difficulties.

General principles for teaching math to children with fragile X again focus on their cognitive strengths and weaknesses. Girls' stronger language skills make auditory explanations of mathematical concepts very important. They may comprehend concrete word problems with meaningful tasks better than they do the nonverbal inputs of numerals, sizes, and shapes.

Boys often require more use of concrete materials. Work with real objects by the child himself may make such concepts as size, order, and shape meaningful. Braden (2000a, 2002a) recommends the use of visual models, patterns, and manipulatives to illustrate concepts such as addition and subtraction.

Clear worksheets, with bold, bright numbers, a limited number of problems, and a liberal use of space are very necessary.

In addressing processing weaknesses of children with fragile X, teachers need to think about visual-spatial and writing problems as part of the math lessons. Clear worksheets, with bold, bright numbers, a limited number of problems, and a liberal use of space are very necessary. The amount to be copied should be monitored when the focus is on math instead of copying or writing. Graph paper or notebook paper turned sideways may be helpful for children who must keep numbers in columns.

Math Curriculum

Functional math is required by all children to gain some levels of independence. A focus on number identification, money, time, and measurement can lead to many applications. For young children and those with more severe disabilities, a focus on number identification and simple computations may be appropriate. Some educators have found "Touch Math" to be effective, as children use tactile strategies with large dots on the numerals to help them remember numbers and values.

Reading and interpreting clocks, calendars and daily planners; following tables and schedules for transportation; interpreting measurements for recipes; and identifying and using money are vital skills for independent living and employment. For example, the use of coins can be presented in this progression:

1. The student recognizes the correct coin when named by the instructor.

2. The student names the coins and comprehends their values.

3. The student combines coins to calculate a given value (e.g., "What coins do you need to make 38 cents?").

The topic of money may lead to combined math, language, and social goals, as the elementary school class plays store or a high school group goes on a shopping expedition.

A focus on the memorization of math facts or multiplication tables might be less necessary than the usage of a calculator to determine the cost of groceries. While children with fragile X may be able to use their good long-term memories to recite a list of math facts, the exercise may not be tied to any higher level of meaningful processing.

Other Academic Areas

Science, social studies, and health may all be classes in which children with fragile X are included in regular education, especially during their elementary school years. Speech-language pathologists and special education teachers find themselves determining what is relevant and appropriate curriculum, adapting that curriculum, pre-teaching vocabulary, assisting with lab experiments, and providing visual aids and real-world examples.

In special education classes, these subjects are also important, especially as they affect functional living areas. Curriculum may center around cooking chemistry, weather, travel and directions, current events, and other areas of interest outside the classroom. Goals regarding reading, writing, and math can all be incorporated into these topical areas with a focus on real world examples and meaningful applications.

Computer Literacy

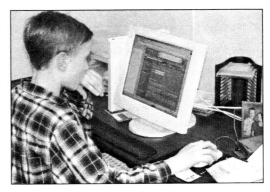

The area of computer literacy cuts across a variety of academic and skill areas and provides excellent leisure skills for many children with fragile X syndrome. Scharfenaker, O'Connor, Stackhouse, Braden, and Gray (2002) find computers to be very important for children with fragile X syndrome for a variety of reasons. They state that computers can help hold attention, give the child time alone without the demands of social interaction, allow for meaningful learning, and help with the production of written language.

Software that addresses pre-academic, academic, language, and recreation/leisure activities can all be integrated into classrooms. Within many software products are a variety of levels, from easy to challenging, so that activities and games may be tailored for the individual child. Computer time can be used as a calming technique or as a reward for completion of other tasks. With headphones and carrels, computer areas provide the small, quiet spaces needed by children with fragile X at various points in their days.

Software may target keyboarding skills or a variety of skills that do not require extensive keyboarding. Keyboarding lessons can be used to focus on letter matching, recognition of letter names, and sequencing of letter combinations. When writing is especially difficult for a child with fragile X, keyboarding provides a more rewarding and less frustrating way to complete written tasks.

Conclusions

Children and adolescents with fragile X syndrome are unique individuals, who perform at a wide range of cognitive levels. Despite their differences, there are many common patterns seen in their learning strengths and weaknesses. Knowledge of the etiology-specific characteristics and application of them to teaching strategies make for most effective academic progress for these students.

chapter 9

Biological Basis

Many readers of this book will focus on the practical suggestions offered in the previous chapters, so why should you be interested in understanding the biological basis of fragile X syndrome? Here are two reasons:

1. With an inherited disease like fragile X syndrome, many questions emerge:

   - Why is there such a large range of expression in the characteristics?
   - Why are boys affected more than girls?
   - Are other family members likely to be affected?
   - What is the probability that a future child will have the disease?
   - How does one diagnose fragile X syndrome?

   While this chapter will not make you an expert in genetic counseling, it will help you understand the issues involved in answering these questions.

2. The story of the cause of fragile X syndrome is one of the most exciting developments in our understanding of complex inherited diseases. As you will see, a picture is emerging that describes this progression:

   - A mutation in the DNA can turn off a gene.
   - The turning off of the gene stops the production of a protein.
   - The lack of the protein blocks normal development of neurons.
   - The limited development of the neurons limits brain activity.
   - The limited brain activity makes it difficult to do math problems.

   In other words, this chapter will explain that Fred failed the math test because one of his ancestors had a cytosine instead of an adenine in a particular spot in the gene that causes fragile X syndrome.

As we fill in the details of the sequence of events outlined above, we discover possibilities where intervention might be used to block the impact of fragile X syndrome. We also develop a model for understanding other diseases that impact cognition and behavior.

Brief History of Genetics

In the 1860s, Gregor Mendel demonstrated that offspring receive half of their genetic information from each parent. With this model, he was able to explain the patterns of inheritance that he saw in garden peas.

In the 1890s, researchers showed that chromosomes are divided up when sperm and eggs are formed. They saw that each egg and sperm receives half of the parent's chromosomes.

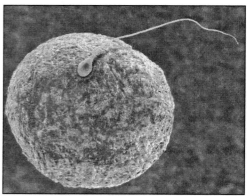

Copyright © Dennis Kunkel Microscopy, Inc.

human egg and sperm

Early in the 1900s, others put these two ideas together and figured out that the genetic information that Mendel studied is located on chromosomes. Work in the 1940s made it clear that it is deoxyribonucleic acid (DNA) in those chromosomes that controls inheritance.

During the next two decades a pattern emerged:

Chromosomes contain DNA,
which controls the synthesis of mRNA,
which controls the synthesis of protein,
which controls physical characteristics.

In other words, the information for how to build and manage the cells of a human being is stored in a person's DNA. A messenger ribonucleic acid (mRNA) copy is made of sections of that DNA. Each molecule of mRNA synthesized, is used to control the assembly of a particular protein. The collection of proteins a cell produces determines what kind of cell will form and what the cell will do. The collection of cells determines the physical characteristics that will be present in the body. So ultimately, DNA controls the physical characteristics.

This overall pattern doesn't explain why a specific change (mutation) in a chromosome can cause the specific physical characteristics of fragile X syndrome. Results of recent studies are helping us tell a more complete story about what causes fragile X syndrome.

Model of Genetic Information

Genetic information is encoded in DNA. The way in which the subunits, *adenine*, *thymine*, *guanine*, and *cytosine* (A, T, G, & C) are arranged, determines whether an egg develops into a human or a pine tree. In a similar way, the letters of the alphabet can be used to describe how to build a kayak or describe how to build a refrigerator.

The DNA in each human cell contains 3 billion pairs of these A, T, G, and C subunits. Since it is hard to imagine 3 billion units of anything, let's compare this to letters of the alphabet. We can put 1500 letters and spaces on a single page and can bind 400 of those pages into a book. Five thousand of those books would contain written text with 3 billion spaces and letters.

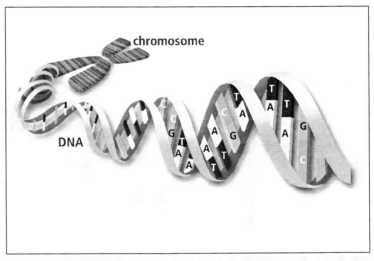

U.S. Department of Energy Human Genome Program (http://www.ornl.gov/hgmis)

In other words, to write out the sequence of A's, T's G's and C's in a single person's DNA would require creating a library of 5000 books. Each microscopic cell in that person contains an identical copy of that library. A change in one of those bases (A, T, G, or C) can result in an inherited disease. In other words, a typographical error (mutation) in one word (codon) on one page (gene) in one of those 5000 books (chromosome) can create misinformation (nonfunctional protein) that confuses the reader (inherited disease).

The following represents 600 of a person's 3,000,000,000 base pairs. The complete sequence of the genetic code for a person would be 5,000,000 times this size.

atctctacacttaagccatatcctctgctccatcaactagtttgccattttgagtaatgggatgaagggtcagcact-
cacagcaagctgcacgcccaacaccatcatcctcttcttccaaaagaaatgcagttctgtttaggacagcaaggt-
gtctggctacaatcctcaggcttccttgtagctatgtgtggtcaggtaacatggtcctagccaatgagatgtaagcag
aaatctactgaatgtagatttctcaatgcagggagagcaagtattttcctgattattattttttaaaggagcagctg-
gcatgtgccttttgcactatgttcttaaacccttttttcctgcataaaatgtaaactcatggtctagagaaggagcagt-
caacttcccagcatgggaatttcaaggaggattagtgggaagaagaaggcgccaccagactacatcctgactgcct
gtctccagacttcttgttacataaaaagaaaaaatgaaataaaataaaataaacccttttacttgtttaagt-
caatattttcagatttaagtgatatatagtcaaatgtaaccagatc

X-Linked Inheritance

Each cell in a human female has two complete sets of chromosomes. Each of her parents gives her one complete set of information on how to assemble a human being. She has one pair of X chromosomes (sex chromosomes) and twenty-two pairs of chromosomes that are not sex chromosomes (autosomes).

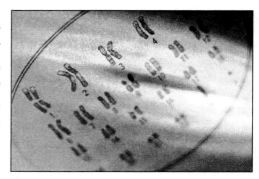

Males also have twenty-two pairs of autosomes and one pair of sex chromosomes. However, for the male, one of those sex chromosomes is a small Y chromosome that he got from his father and the other is an X chromosome that he received from his mother. The Y chromosome sets in motion the development of male characteristics but has very few genes.

As a result, inheritance of X-linked genes differs between males and females. Males get all of their X-linked genes from their mothers, while females receive one collection of X-linked genes from each parent.

Inheritance of Hemophilia

Before we discuss the complex system of inheritance in fragile X syndrome, let's review the inheritance of a better-known X-linked disease in humans, hemophilia. Most people are able to produce a protein clotting factor, which causes their blood to coagulate when it comes in contact with oxygen in the air. As a result, when they get a cut, the leakage is blocked by the formation of a clot. Persons with hemophilia will continue to bleed from a cut; they don't make the protein clotting factor and as a result, the blood does not coagulate.

This disease is inherited in a fairly straightforward way. There are three versions (genotypes) of females with respect to hemophilia.

> ✳ Females with two copies of the dominant version of the gene will have blood that can coagulate, since both produce the clotting factor.
>   • X^H X^H — **Female:** *Non-affected*

* Females with one copy producing the clotting factor and one that doesn't, will not exhibit uncontrolled bleeding, since one working copy is enough. As a result, clotting is dominant over not clotting.
  * X^H X^h — **Female:** *Non-affected carrier*

* The only females to express hemophilia, receive a nonfunctional copy of the gene from each of their parents.
  * X^h X^h — **Female:** *Hemophiliac (rare)*

Males come in two versions (genotypes) with respect to hemophilia:

* Most males have the version of the gene that leads to the ability to clot blood.
  * X^H Y — **Male:** *Non-affected*

* The rest of the males will express uncontrolled bleeding because they don't have the ability to make the clotting factor.
  * X^h Y — **Male:** *Hemophiliac*

Some general patterns that emerge with hemophilia are:

* Females must get a defective copy from each parent to express the disorder.
* Males can only get the disorder from their mothers.
* A carrier female does not express the disorder.
* Each son of a carrier female has a 50% chance of being affected.

Inheritance of Fragile X Syndrome

The fragile X mental retardation (FMR1) gene controls the synthesis of the fragile X mental retardation (FMR) protein. The absence of the FMR protein causes fragile X syndrome. While the pattern of inheritance of the FMR1 gene superficially resembles that of hemophilia, it is much more complex. In addition, as you will see later, the FMR1 gene occurs in many different versions.

* A female who has two copies of the regular fmr1 gene will not have fragile X syndrome.
  * X^{fmr1} X^{fmr1} — **Female:** *Non-affected*

✳ A female who has one copy of the regular fmr1 gene and one of the full mutant version may exhibit some of the characteristics of fragile X syndrome or none of them. This range in expression will be discussed later. (Since the mutant version shows up in the presence of the standard version, we say the mutation is *dominant*. We use uppercase letters for the dominant version [allele] and lowercase letters for the recessive version.)

• X^{fmr1} X^{FMR1} — **Female:** *May have fragile X symptoms*

✳ It would be unusual for a female to have two copies of the full mutant version of the gene. As will be discussed later, children can only get the full mutation from their mothers, so a female cannot get a full mutation from each parent.

• X^{FMR1} X^{FMR1} — **Female:** *Fragile X (rare or non-existent)*

✳ A male with one regular fmr1 gene will not have fragile X syndrome.

• X^{fmr1} Y — **Male:** *Non-affected*

✳ A male with the full mutation will probably exhibit a number of the characteristics of fragile X syndrome; however, it is also possible that he will have few symptoms.

• X^{FMR1} Y — **Male:** *Probably has fragile X symptoms*

Protein Production in Fragile X Syndrome and Hemophilia

Both hemophilia and fragile X syndrome follow the general pattern of inheritance described on page 118. For each, the DNA in the chromosome contains a gene that controls the synthesis of messenger RNA (mRNA). The mRNA contains coded information for how to make a particular protein. When the protein is made, the parts of the body that need that protein are able to function normally.

We can tell what the role of the hemophilia gene is by looking at someone who doesn't have the protein the gene codes for. When the gene has a mutation and the cells are unable to make the protein clotting factor, or make a clotting factor that doesn't work, a cut will continue to bleed. When the clotting factor is present in a functional form, the blood will clot to stop the bleeding if the person gets cut. Since the protein is needed in the circulatory system, not in individual cells, we can easily replace the missing clotting factor in a person who has hemophilia.

The FMR (fragile X mental retardation) protein produced by the FMR1 gene plays roles in many parts of the body. We know this because a person who cannot produce this specific protein may exhibit abnormal development in the heart, feet, testicles, brain, and other parts of the body. When the FMR protein is present, one typically finds normal development in those areas.

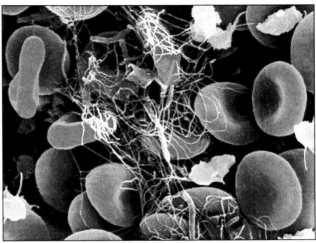

Copyright © Dennis Kunkel Microscopy, Inc.

red blood cells trapped in a fibrin blood clot

Since the FMR protein is needed in a variety of tissues at different times in development and at various levels of concentration, replacing the missing protein is likely to be more difficult than replacing the clotting factor in someone who has hemophilia. This difficulty has been demonstrated in studies of mice that have defective FMR1 genes (Bakker et al., 2000; Peier et al., 2000).

Gene Mutations in Fragile X Syndrome and Hemophilia

Although somewhat of an oversimplification, one could say that variations in the clotting gene fall into two categories: either the gene codes for a functional protein or it doesn't. As a result, one either inherits a working or a nonworking gene from a parent. New mutations, or changes in the DNA coding for the clotting factor, are rare: the functional and non-functional versions of this gene get passed from generation to generation with few modifications.

In contrast, the variations in the FMR1 gene can be divided into three categories, standard, premutation, and full mutation. Each of those three categories has many variants. Furthermore, the gene can change or mutate from generation to generation.

Standard Version of the FMR1 Gene

There is a section of the FMR1 gene that has a series of CGG (cytosine, guanine, guanine) repeats. Most people have 6-55 copies of the CGG repeat and do not exhibit fragile X syndrome. They will pass on a similar number of repeats to their children and grandchildren. An FMR1 gene with 55 or fewer repeats is usually stable from generation to generation.

The following sequence is from one individual's FMR1 gene. Since this person has 19 copies of the CGG repeat, this is the standard version.

agcagcgcgcatgcgcgcgctcccaggccacttgaagagagagggcggggccgaggggctgagcccgcggggggaggg
aacagcgttgatcacgtgacgtggtttcagtgtttacacccgcagcgggccggggttcggcctcagtcaggcgctcagctccg
tttcggtttcacttccggtggagggccgcctctgagcgggcggcggccgacggcgagcgcgggcggcggcggtgacgga
ggcgccgctgccagggggcgtgcggcagcg**cggcggcggcggcggcggcggcggcggcgg**a**gg**cg
gcggcggcggcggcggcggcggcggctgggcctcgagcgcccgcagcccacctctcgggggcgggctcccg
gcgctagcagggctgaagagaagatggaggagctggtggtggaagtgcggggctccaatggcgctttctacaaggtacttgg
ctctagggcaggccccatctttccctccctttcttcttggtgtcggcgggaggcaggcccggggccctcttcccgagcaccgcg
cctgggtgccagggcacgctcggcgggatgttgttgggagggaaggactggacttggggcctgttggaagcccctctccgact
ccgagaggccctagcgcctatcgaaatgagagaccagcgaggagagggttctctttcggcgccgagccccgccggggtgag
ctggggatgggcgagggccggcggcaggtactagagccgggcgggaagggccgaaatcggc

This series of CGG repeats has an AGG in the middle. Periodic AGG's among the CGG's contribute additional stability in the FMR1 gene, decreasing even more the possibility of having a child with a different number of repeats than observed in the parent (Zhong, Yang, Dobkin, & Brown, 1995). These AGG's appear to serve as anchors, preventing "slippage" when the DNA is copied during cell division (Pearson et al., 1998). In the absence of those anchors, there seems to be a slight increase in the probability that the offspring will have a number of repeats that is larger or smaller than that of the parent.

Premutation of the FMR1 Gene

Some people have 55-200 CGG repeats in their FMR1 gene. This is defined as a premutation because it is unstable and is likely to result in a full mutation in a subsequent generation. Most of those with the premutation (both male and female) will experience few or no effects from the mutated gene.

All of the daughters of a male with the premutation will receive the premutation from the father; the number of repeats may be larger or smaller in the daughter but it will not be in excess of 200 (Nolin et al., 1996). All of the sons of a male with the premutation will receive a Y chromosome from their father; these sons will not get fragile X syndrome since the FMR1 gene is on the X chromosome.

A female with the premutation, has one X chromosome with the premutation and another with the standard version. Each of her children will receive one of her X chromosomes. If the child receives the X chromosome with the standard version, the child will not have fragile X and will not have children with fragile X.

If the child receives the X chromosome that had the premutation, the number of repeats is likely to be larger than observed in the mother. If the mother has 100-200 repeats, she is very likely to pass on more than 200 repeats to that child, resulting in a full mutation (Nolin et al., 2003).

Full Mutation of the FMR1 Gene

If a person has more than 200 CGG repeats, the full mutation is set in motion. The FMR1 gene is turned off, no working mRNA copy is made of the gene, and as a result, no FMR protein is synthesized. These individuals will have the physical and behavioral characteristics of fragile X syndrome.

Females with one copy of the full mutation will pass either the X chromosome with the full mutation or the X chromosome that does not have the mutation to each of their children. As a result, each child has a 50/50 chance of getting the full mutation.

Males with the full mutation do not usually father children. Those who have children will pass on a Y chromosome to their sons; they cannot give any version of the FMR1 gene to their sons since it is on the X chromosome. Curiously, they will pass on a premutation (reduced number of repeats) to their daughters (Gane & Cronister, 2002).

Testing for Fragile X

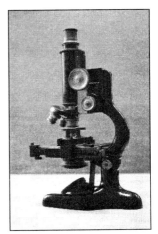

The only tool available in the 1980s and 1990s to diagnose fragile X syndrome was a cytogenetic test in which one looked for abnormally shaped X chromosomes. While this test is still useful for detecting a variety of chromosome abnormalities, it is no longer a primary tool for fragile X identification (Gane & Cronister, 2002).

As discussed in this chapter, two factors play significant roles in the expression of fragile X. The first is the number of CGG repeats; we can determine this number with the polymerase chain reaction (PCR) test. PCR is a method of copying a small section of the DNA over and over. By making copies of the section of the FMR1 gene with repeats, we can precisely identify the number of repeats present. This works particularly well to differentiate those with the stable number of repeats (up to 55) from those at the lower end of the premutation range (55-200). It is technically more difficult to use PCR for analysis of those with a full mutation (above 200 repeats), and some females with a full mutation will not be identified (Brown, 2002).

The second factor (discussed below) determining the expression of fragile X is methylation of the DNA, typically present in those with more than 200 repeats. Southern blot analysis is used to test for methylation and to identify those with large numbers of repeats (Tarleton, 2003). Southern blot analysis is more expensive than PCR analysis (Brown, 2002).

A fourth approach to testing is to test directly for the presence of the FMR protein. Since hair roots typically produce significant amounts of FMR protein, its absence can be readily determined by an inexpensive protein analysis (Willemsen et al., 1999). This test will not identify those with the premutation, only those with the full mutation.

Turning off the FMR1 Gene

Cells utilize a variety of methods to regulate levels of different proteins in a cell. Each cell of the body has the same library of information, yet the kidney makes a different set of proteins than those produced in liver cells. One of the regulatory methods is methylation, in which an enzyme can add methyl groups (a carbon and three hydrogens) to a specific part of the DNA. This appears to make that

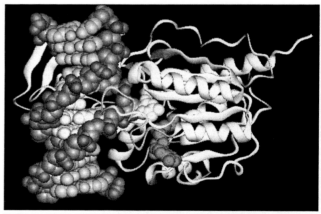

Courtesy of Richard J. Roberts, New England Biolabs

model of an enzyme (right) methylating a DNA molecule

particular region of DNA unavailable and as a result, an mRNA copy cannot be made. With no mRNA copy, the protein coded for by that part of the DNA, will not be assembled (Holliday, 1993).

Earlier we stated that when there are more than 200 CGG repeats, the FMR1 gene is turned off. The presence of the full mutation (more than 200 repeats) sets in motion the methylation of the specific section of DNA that regulates the FMR1 gene. Someone with more than 200 repeats fails to make the FMR protein, not because of the repeats, but because the repeats cause the methylation of the regulatory site for the FMR1 gene.

This suggests that individuals with 55-200 repeats should have no methylation and therefore no impact from the premutation. In general that is true; however, analysis of these individuals shows that as the number of repeats increases, the FMR protein levels go down somewhat (Kenneson, Zhang, Hagedorn, & Warren, 2001; Tassone, Hagerman, Chamberlain, & Hagerman, 2000). Curiously, the levels of mRNA coding for the FMR protein go up (Tassone, Hagerman, Taylor et al., 2000). These individuals are overproducing the mRNA, but even with extra mRNA, are not quite able to maintain the normal level of FMR protein.

Apparently there are two mechanisms that turn off the FMR1 gene: one mechanism exhibited by those with the premutation, and the second mechanism, methylation, activated by the presence of more than 200 CGG copies.

Variation in FMR Protein Levels

Typically, a female puts one complete set of her chromosomes into an egg, making it *haploid*, and a male puts a haploid set of his chromosomes into each sperm. The fertilized egg gets two sets of chromosomes, one from each parent, making it *diploid*. Each time that cell divides, it produces two cells that each have two complete sets of genetic information. Since the mechanism for copying DNA is very precise, each cell in the human body should get an identical copy of the library of genetic information. Sometimes it doesn't work that way.

FMR Protein Levels in Mosaic Males

In a male with the full mutation on the X chromosome, one would expect to find no FMR protein; all of his cells should have an X chromosome with a nonfunctional FMR1 gene and a Y chromosome that does not carry the FMR1 gene. This is what we do find in many males with the full mutation.

There are, however, some males with the full mutation who are capable of synthesizing limited FMR protein. These males are mosaic, having two kinds of cells: some with the premutation and others with the full mutation. The expansion of the CGG repeats takes place after the fertilized egg has begun to divide. When there is already a ball of cells formed, a switch is thrown and some cells have an expansion in the FMR1 gene, while others do not. As a result, some of the cells retain the premutation that the mother had, and others expand to the full mutation. In these mosaic individuals, we find that there are various levels of FMR protein and various levels of impact from fragile X syndrome. The level of FMR protein expression accounts for some of the level of total development in males with fragile X (Bailey, Hatton, Tassone, Skinner, & Taylor, 2001). In other words, some of these males are not as severely affected as males in which no FMR protein is synthesized.

X Chromosome Inactivation in Females

The presence of two X chromosomes in females and only one in males presents a potential general problem for all mammals, including humans. For each protein that is coded for by an X-linked gene, females have two genes and males only one. That could lead to females overproducing those proteins or males underproducing them. Cells in mammals have a simple solution for that problem. Females only use one of the two X chromosomes in each of their cells (Lyon, 1962). They inactivate the other X chromosome by methylating it as discussed above. This way, males and females each have one working X chromosome in each cell, equalizing the dosage of proteins coded for by the X chromosome.

FMR Protein Levels in Females

In females with the full mutation on one of the X chromosomes, one would expect to find a mixture of cells, some producing FMR protein and others producing no FMR protein. This is a possible explanation for the fact that females typically express a milder version of the symptoms of fragile X when compared to males. While some of a female's cells are using the X chromosome with the defective FMR1 gene, other cells are using the X chromosome that is capable of producing FMR protein.

This also might explain why there is such a wide variation in expression of fragile X symptoms among females. The ratio of cells with a working copy of the gene to those with no working copy (activation ratio) varies depending on how many cells were fortunate enough to inactivate the X chromosome with the nonworking FMR1 gene. In one family, one sister displays many of the characteristics of a male with the full mutation; most of her tested cells have inactivated the working FMR1 gene. Her sister is only mildly affected; most of her tested cells have inactivated the mutated FMR1 gene (Heine-Suner et al., 2003).

The location of the cells is also critical. Imagine that an area of the body that normally produces a lot of FMR protein, such as the brain, has a lot of cells that do make the FMR protein, and a tissue that has no need for FMR protein has a lot of cells that are incapable of making the protein. In such a case, the nonfunctioning FMR1 gene should not have any impact on the cells that don't need it and the cells that need the FMR protein, have a working copy.

Role of FMR Protein

FMR protein has been shown to play a role in regulating the synthesis of specific proteins (Laggerbauer, Ostareck, Keidel, Ostareck-Lederer, & Fischer, 2001). Thus, the absence of FMR protein has the potential to interrupt the normal regulation of other proteins or enzymes that play important roles in the brain and other parts of the body.

If the FMR protein were required for the regulation of all protein synthesis, its absence would trigger death. If the FMR protein were required only for regulation of the synthesis of relatively unimportant proteins, we would never notice its absence. Since the absence of FMR protein triggers significant problems, but not death, its role is somewhere in the middle of those two extremes.

Regulation of Neuron Development

Mice without a functioning FMR1 gene do not make the FMR protein and as a result, their brains do not develop normally (Nimchinsky, Oberlander, & Svoboda, 2001).

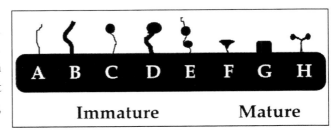

Irwin, S. A., Patel, B., Idupulapati, M., Harris, J. B., Crisostomo, R. A., Larsen, B. P., et al. (2001). Abnormal dendritic spine characteristics in the temporal and visual cortices of patients with fragile-X syndrome: a quantitative examination. Copyright © 2001 Wiley-Liss, Inc. Reprinted by permission of Wiley-Liss, Inc., a subsidiary of John Wiley & Sons, Inc.

spine morphology categories

Neurons have branches (dendrites) through which they communicate with other neurons. During normal development of dendrites in the brain, the dendrite sends out numerous spines that are potential connections to other neurons. In the immature mouse, these spines have immature shapes. If the mouse lives in a simple environment where there is little stimulation, the spines remain numerous and immature as the mouse grows older (Churchill et al., 2002).

If the mouse lives in a complex environment where there is stimulating activity, two changes will occur. The spines will take on a different (mature) shape, and there will be a pruning of the spines. The mature neuron will have fewer dendritic spines, but those remaining will be mature connections to other neurons (Churchill et al., 2002), such as those in the control individual in the illustration.

If the mouse lives in a stimulating environment but has a defective FMR1 gene and doesn't make FMR protein, the spines remain numerous and immature (Comery et al., 1997) as illustrated by the individual with fragile X in the illustration. Thus, the absence of FMR protein results in the failure of neurons in the brain to make appropriate connections to other neurons.

Fragile X   Control

Irwin, S. A., Patel, B., Idupulapati, M., Harris, J. B., Crisostomo, R. A., Larsen, B. P., et al. (2001). Abnormal dendritic spine characteristics in the temporal and visual cortices of patients with fragile-X syndrome: a quantitative examination. Copyright © 2001 Wiley-Liss, Inc. Reprinted by permission of Wiley-Liss, Inc., a subsidiary of John Wiley & Sons, Inc.

human dendrites with spines

Regulation of Brain Activity

Susan Rivera and colleagues (2002) have studied the way in which brain activity is correlated with functional skills. They take MRI scans of people while they are trying to answer questions in order to determine where the brain is active during problem solving.

Children who do not have fragile X syndrome are given math problems in which two numbers are added. They are asked if the stated answer is correct. Immediately, the MRI shows activity in a number of areas of the brain. If they are asked to check the addition of three numbers, the activity in those areas increases, and new areas become visibly active.

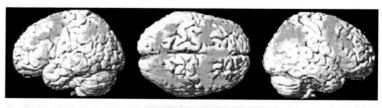

Courtesy of Allan Reiss, School of Medicine, Stanford University

control subject during a memory task

Children with fragile X syndrome are given the same math problems. When adding two numbers, there is less brain activity than is seen in children who don't have fragile X syndrome. When the children with fragile X are asked to add three numbers, the brain pattern resembles that seen when they are adding two numbers.

. . . when the task gets more difficult, children without fragile X use more areas of the brain and in general use the brain more intensely.

In other words, when the task gets more difficult, children without fragile X use more areas of the brain and in general use the brain more intensely. Children with fragile X approach simple and hard math problems with the same low level of brain activity. Similar results were found when studying visuospatial working memory in children with fragile X (Kwon et al., 2001).

Cause of Fragile X Syndrome

So why did Fred fail the mathematics quiz? He failed it because one of his ancestors had a long series of CGGs in the FMR1 gene, uninterrupted by an AGG. The box provides a summary of all the processes that lead up to the simple failure of a child with fragile X to complete a mathematics problem.

For Lack of an AGG, the Math Quiz Was Failed

Lack of AGGs among the CGGs elicits

abnormal alignment of DNA,

which causes slippage during DNA replication,

resulting in increased CGGs in offspring,

triggering methlation of a regulatory site,

which blocks normal synthesis of mRNA, and,

therefore, doesn't allow production of FMRP protein,

setting in motion unregulated synthesis of other proteins in dendrites,

causing abnormal development of spines,

preventing typical wiring of the brain,

blocking usual patterns of brain activation,

creating difficulties in adding three numbers.

So What Can We Do?

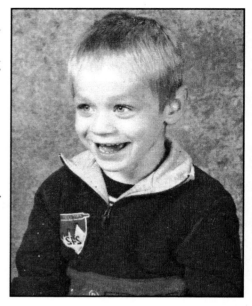

The box on page 131 describes the biological sequence of events leading to a problem in doing mathematics. Of course, the story doesn't end there. As you have seen in the previous chapters, we have discovered a wide range of interventions to address the physical, cognitive, and sensory impacts of fragile X. Most of those interventions address the final step in the sequence. In other words, they do not attempt to target the biological causes of fragile X; they target the symptoms that result from the sequence of biological events. In many cases, addressing those symptoms can be an effective response to limit the impact of fragile X syndrome.

Our current understanding of the series of biological dominoes opens up new possibilities for intervention. In addition to the interventions that address the end result, we can begin to focus on earlier steps in the sequence. In the next chapter, we will identify areas of future development that build on our understanding of the biological causes of fragile X syndrome.

chapter 10 Future Directions

Behavioral, Educational, and Therapeutic Treatment

For years, we have explored ways to address the impact of fragile X on individuals. Most of that focus has been to target the specific symptoms that result from the syndrome. For example, a negative behavior may have a biological basis, but as you have seen in the previous chapters, we have learned that it is possible to modify, refocus, or prevent that behavior using behavioral, educational, and therapeutic techniques.

The continuing research in this area will be critical for several reasons. While there are intriguing possibilities regarding interventions to block the biological impact of fragile X, the realization of those possibilities may be years away. Those solutions may have costs that make them prohibitive except for a few individuals. In addition, even if we find biological answers for fragile X syndrome, it is unlikely that we will find a perfect solution that doesn't need the support that comes from treatment of symptoms.

Through the efforts of many people, Congress passed the Children's Health Act of 2000. One component of that was the establishment of Fragile X Treatment and Research Centers at three different locations: the University of Washington, the University of North Carolina, and Baylor College of Medicine. The centers are to "conduct and support basic and biomedical research into the detection and treatment of fragile X" (Children's Health Act of 2000, 2000).

Medical Treatment

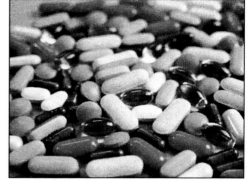

In this book, we have not discussed medications, but an extensive discussion of those issues has been summarized by Randi Hagerman (2002a) and is available on the National Fragile X Foundation Web site: www.fragilex.org.

We have learned a lot about the role that medications can play, particularly in modifying activity in the brain. As with treatment of symptoms through behavioral and educational methods, we will continue to explore the treatment of symptoms with medications.

Some of the new research is focusing on medical treatment that will address the mechanism of fragile X, not just the resulting symptoms. One example is research on *ampakines*. This family of molecules increases production of brain-derived neurotrophic factor (BDNF), which in turn contributes to a reduction in dendrite spine number and length (Lauterborn, 2003). In theory, this has the potential to correct one of the abnormalities observed in humans and mice with fragile X syndrome.

Research on ampakines is progressing on two fronts. One of the ampakines has been approved for testing in humans; a clinical study of 26 human subjects who have fragile X or autism is currently underway (Berry-Kravis, 2003). The mechanism of action of a more powerful ampakine is being tested in rodents (Lauterborn, 2003; Lauterborn et al., 2003).

Folic Acid

Some of the early research on fragile X suggested that fragile X might be cured with a simple medication. As was discussed earlier, Lubs (1969) noticed an unusual constriction in the X chromosomes of several patients who were mentally retarded. Over the next decade, some researchers confirmed his observation while others found only normal-looking chromosomes in similar individuals. Sutherland (1977) showed that in order to see this fragile-looking chromosome, one needed to culture the cells in a particular type of growth medium. He later demonstrated that the reason the growth medium triggered the appearance of defective chromosomes was that the growth medium was missing folic acid (Sutherland, 1979).

This suggested a possible nutritional cause of fragile X. If the lack of folic acid caused chromosomes from someone with fragile X to grow oddly in the test tube, perhaps a shortage of folic acid caused the symptoms of fragile X in that person. If the problem was reversible, then giving folic acid to someone with fragile X might block the symptoms. Alternatively, if the problems were not reversible, it might at least be possible to prevent future cases of fragile X by giving folic acid supplements during pregnancy.

Women planning a pregnancy are encouraged to take folic acid supplements, but that is because it has been shown to decrease the incidence of neural tube defects, not that it prevents fragile X syndrome.

Since then, we have discovered that folic acid is not a simple cure for fragile X syndrome. Women planning a pregnancy are encouraged to take folic acid supplements, but that is because it has been shown to decrease the incidence of neural tube defects, not that it prevents fragile X syndrome (Lucock, 2000). Some individuals with fragile X do experience limited benefits from folic acid medication but it does not appear to help others (R. Hagerman, 2002a).

Just Add FMR Protein

The discovery of the FMR protein suggested another possibility: if the body fails to make a specific protein, perhaps we could just replace it. It is important to understand that it is not the lack of general proteins that causes fragile X syndrome. One could think of proteins as tools. If we need a particular screwdriver to adjust an engine so it will run, having a warehouse full of hammers, rakes, and other tools will be of no help. Similarly, feeding someone lots of eggs and tofu will give the person lots of protein, but not the particular protein that is missing in a person with fragile X.

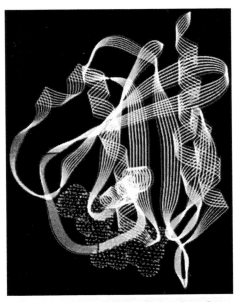

U.S. Department of Energy Human Genome Program
(http://www.ornl.gov/hgmis)

model of the ras protein that regulates cell growth

Inside the Cells

Perhaps one could find a way to produce the FMR protein and give it to persons with fragile X. After all, we give insulin to people with diabetes, growth hormone to those who don't produce it, and clotting factor to people with hemophilia. In each of these cases, the

Future Directions

substance we provide travels through the circulatory system before it plays its particular role. It is relatively easy, therefore, to determine if the blood has an appropriate amount; if not, we can supplement by adding the missing substance to the blood.

FMR protein stays in the cells that produce it and carries out its role in those same cells. Presumably, one would need to add the protein to thousands or millions of individual cells in just the right amount. How do you get it into the cells?

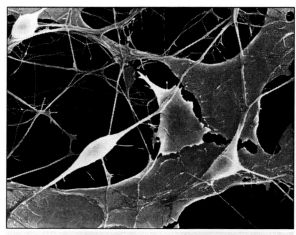

Copyright © Dennis Kunkel Microscopy, Inc.

pyramidal neurons

One couldn't simply add the FMR protein to the diet. If added to one's food, most of the protein would be digested and its subunits (amino acids) reassembled into new proteins. Injecting the FMR protein into individual cells is not a simple task.

Virus Proteins Can Help

If you inject the protein into the blood, it is unable to get across the blood-brain barrier and unable to get inside a cell. However, it has been discovered that some viruses have the equivalent of a key. A small section (domain) of one of their proteins (a translocatory protein) has the ability to help slip the protein across a membrane. HIV that causes AIDS and herpes simplex virus each have a protein that has a protein transduction domain (PTD) that aids in translocation across membranes of cells. That small domain can be attached to a different protein and help it get across the membrane. Recent research is helping us understand the mechanism by which these PTDs work (Leifert & Whitton, 2003; Lundberg, Wikström, & Johansson, 2003)

This offers us a way in which to get proteins across the blood-brain barrier and across cell membranes into neurons. It would not be a one-time treatment, since the cells would not be making their own protein, and the protein would be broken down fairly quickly. We would need to treat the person regularly with additional protein. We might not need to worry about getting too much in, because if a cell got too much, it would soon dissipate.

We don't know if the protein will survive long enough in the blood to get to the cells in the brain, and we're not actually sure the protein will work if it gets there, since it has the attached PTD (P. Hagerman, 2000).

In the Right Cells

Even if we get the FMR protein into cells, we need to get it into the right cells. In individuals who do not have fragile X syndrome, the protein is not equally distributed. It is found at high levels in neurons but low levels in the nearby glial cells. It is found at high levels in spermatogonia (cells in the testes that have not yet begun the formation of sperm) but not in the more mature cells nor in the nearby helper Sertoli cells (Devys, Lutz, Rouyer, Bellocq, & Mandel, 1993). So what happens if we flood the brain or the entire body with FMR protein? It may help the cells that need it, but it could be toxic to cells that normally do not produce it (P. Hagerman, 2000).

Fine Tune the Existing System

If fragile X is caused by methylation that blocks a regulatory site on the FMR1 gene, why not remove the block? There are chemicals that remove the methylation from DNA or that prevent it from being added to DNA.

One difficulty is that while the methylation is bad for the FMR1 gene, it is essential for other genes in the cell. If a lock in the house doesn't work because it has glue in it, you can't simply spray the entire house with something that dissolves glue. It's true that you would open up the lock, but you might also loosen glue in many other places in the house. If you add a chemical that removes methylation from the DNA, you might make it possible to synthesize FMR protein, but you might also unblock many other genes that ought to remain blocked.

Attempts to reactivate the FMR1 gene in tissue taken from men with fragile X syndrome have resulted in no reactivation (Coffee, Zhang, Warren, & Reines, 1999) or limited reactivation (Chiurazzi et al., 1999). Since these studies were done in tissue culture, it was not possible to look for side effects.

Correct the Translation Problem

While there is evidence that methylation turns off the FMR1 gene, there is also evidence, particularly in persons with the premutation, that the gene is being copied into messenger RNA but that the message doesn't work well. There are a number of strategies that might lead to enhancing the utilization of these messages (P. Hagerman, 2002).

Gene Therapy

A more permanent solution would be to attempt repairs in the cells that have the FMR1 mutation. Gene therapy typically focuses on correcting or compensating for defects in somatic (body) cells, not in reproductive cells. Tinkering with the reproductive cells that will be involved in producing the next generation raises moral and ethical questions that societies have not yet resolved. This discussion, then, will be about ways to affect the person with fragile X syndrome, not ways to repair the gene for future generations.

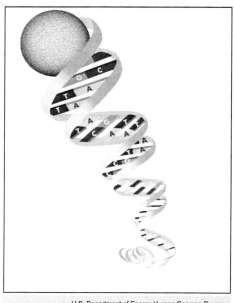

U.S. Department of Energy Human Genome Program
(http://www.ornl.gov/hgmis)

Since 1988, the Recombinant DNA Advisory Committee of the National Institutes of Health has reviewed nearly 600 proposals to do clinical trials (none focused on fragile X) involving human gene transfer (Office of Biotechnology Activities, 2003). Nevertheless, there are no licensed gene therapy products available in the U.S. at this time (Grilley & Gee, 2003).

The initial excitement about human gene transfer was dealt a serious blow with the death of Jesse Gelsinger in 1999 as a result of a gene therapy experiment (Stolberg, 1999). Still, researchers continue to look for safe ways to make genetic repairs in human cells (Rubanyi, 2001).

Replace the FMR1 Gene

Perhaps one could add a working FMR1 gene to the cell. To accomplish that, there are many decisions that need to be made. Do you replace the defective gene with a working one or just add a working one? If the defective one is simply not working, one can ignore it. However, if it is doing bad things, we need to get rid of it.

Obviously, it is much easier to add a gene to the cell if we don't at the same time need to remove the original copy of the gene. As discussed in Chapter 9, removing it would be the equivalent of finding a particular page in a library and destroying it.

One model for how the FMR1 gene works is that the problems associated with fragile X are all because the gene is turned off. In that case, the only thing we need to do is add a working copy; there is no need to get rid of the nonworking copy. If the mutant gene is doing bad things and needs removal, the task is more complicated.

Add a Working FMR1 Gene

For an inserted functional FMR1 gene to successfully address fragile X, it would need to remain unmethylated. If the methylation triggered by the CGG expansion causes methylation of all FMR1 genes in the cell, an inserted working copy will be turned off.

The inserted copy would need to be under cell type control. Many cells in the body do not use their FMR1 gene. If we insert working FMR1 genes into many types of cells and they all use it, it may be helpful to those cells that need it and harmful to those that do not.

Add a Gene or Add a Chromosome?

The next decision is whether to insert the new gene into an existing chromosome or to add it as part of a new chromosome. To use the analogy from Chapter 9, does one insert a new page into an existing book or does one add a new book to the library?

If we inserted a new page into an existing book, it could cause problems. What if we inserted a page with instructions for making brass cleaner into the middle of a cake recipe? Anyone attempting to make the cake would create a toxic product.

If we inserted the working FMR1 gene randomly into a chromosome, we might disrupt another gene. Destroying that gene's ability to work would probably not cause a big problem since it might only affect that gene in 1 out of a million cells. However, many genes play a role in regulating cell division. If we insert DNA into the middle of one of those oncogenes, that one in a million could create a malignancy.

The alternative is to insert a new chromosome that leaves intact the rest of the other chromosomes (Lipps et al., 2003).

How to Get DNA Into Cells

One method of getting the DNA in cells is to inject it directly. An electrical impulse (electroporation) can make cells permeable to DNA and allow them to absorb DNA directly. This has been done to experimentally inject DNA into the synovial membrane in rat knees (Ohashi et al., 2002), and into human skin cells that were grafted onto mouse skin (L. Zhang, Nolan, Kreitschitz, & Rabussay, 2002).

Viral Vectors

Another strategy is to use an existing system that injects DNA into cells. Viruses are protein-wrapped packages of DNA or RNA. They have no ability to grow or reproduce on their own. They must take over control of animal, plant or bacterial cells and use the invaded cells' machinery and raw materials to make new viruses. They do this by injecting their DNA or RNA into a cell. The injected material has the ability to override the normal functioning of the cell so that it is now controlled by the virus.

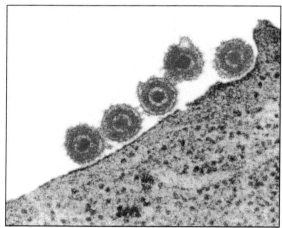

Copyright © Dennis Kunkel Microscopy, Inc.

herpes simplex virus

Fortunately, the ability of viruses to inject DNA and the ability of that DNA to take over control of the cell are under separate control. In other words, we can create hybrid viruses that still retain the ability to inject DNA, but instead of containing DNA that takes control of the invaded cell, they contain DNA from a gene we want to insert into the cell. This way, they serve as vectors to transfer in a working gene without causing a disease.

One such vector is the adenovirus that normally causes upper respiratory tract infections in humans. We can remove the genes that allow it to cause disease, and insert a human gene. Experiments to date with using such viruses have had mixed results. It was an experiment using an adenovirus vector that resulted in the death of Jesse Gelsinger (Stolberg, 1999). New technologies are being developed to target the viruses to particular cells while avoiding infecting other cells that cause significant side effects (Barnett, Crews, & Douglas, 2002).

Non-Viral Vectors

In order to avoid some of the problems associated with viral vectors, researchers have wrapped a gene in a package of molecules that is designed to cross the blood-brain barrier and fuse with brain cells. *Luciferase* is the enzyme that causes fireflies to light up, and researchers demonstrated that they could inject the gene for luciferase, wrapped in a molecular package, into the blood of a monkey. This fake virus then selectively crossed from the blood into the neurons of the brain and produce luciferase (Y. Zhang, Schlachetzki, & Pardridge, 2003). The gene did not remain permanently in the cells; the production of the new protein dropped to 50% within 6 days.

Next Steps

What we have learned about the biological basis of fragile X syndrome offers possibilities for treatment in the future. Researchers in this field have become very excited about the doors they see opening; however, we must approach this discussion with a caution. A researcher may celebrate the discovery of a step in the regulation of protein synthesis by the FMR protein and look years down the road to the day when her discovery contributes to a solution. A family member who works with someone with fragile X syndrome may have a different perspective. He may want to know how the discovery will impact his child in the coming months.

We also do not know how reversible some of fragile X characteristics are. There may be a critical point after which the FMR protein's ability to reverse things is limited. In other words, it may be that the FMR protein plays a critical role in embryonic development or in the first few years of life. Adding the FMR protein after that may not be able to repair the damage that was done; nevertheless, it is possible that if we are able to get the FMR protein into the right cells in the right amount, at the right time, we may partially or completely reverse the impact that the lack of FMR protein has had on an individual. Recently, researchers inserted a working FMR1 gene into the cells of a mouse whose cells did not have a working FMR1 gene. These mice do produce the FMR protein in their cells, but the mice demonstrated only limited reversal of the characteristics seen in mice with fragile X syndrome (Bakker et al., 2000; Peier et al., 2000).

In the meantime, educators, therapists, researchers, physicians, and parents are working together to maximize the potential of children and adults with fragile X syndrome.

Photographic & Illustration Credits

Cover Image: *Fragile X* by Achille Ghidoni

The cover image, *Fragile X*, is a copy of a 30 x 40 cm oil on canvas painting created by Achille Ghidoni in 1996. It was used on the cover of *Genetica Generale e Umana* (Vol. II) written by De Carli, L., Boncinelli, E., Danieli, G. A., & Larizza, L. (1998) and published in Padova, Italy by Piccin. In 2003, the original painting was displayed as part of an art exhibit in Naples, Italy, celebrating the 50th anniversary of the discovery of the structure of DNA. It was previously shown at two exhibitions in Italy and used on the poster for a fragile X workshop in Milano.

Achille Ghidoni recently retired from his positions as Professor of Genetics in the Department of Structural and Functional Biology and Rector's Delegate for International Relations at the University of Insubria in Varese, Italy. Previously he was at the University of Milano. As a result of the painting he has done in his spare time, his artistry has been featured in 10 personal exhibitions in Italy, Germany, and France. Many images from his paintings have been used as covers in scientific journals and books on medicine, biology, and biotechnology. Other works he has painted can be seen on the Web at:

* http://ftp.sunet.se/pub/pictures/art/
* http://www.tigem.it/science&art/Ghidoni/ghidoni.html
* http://q-consulting.mine.nu/cdg/
* http://digilander.libero.it/regre/ghidoni/

Additional Images

Images on pages 125, 134, and 143 are copyrighted © 2003 Dale Fast.

The image on page 120 is copyrighted © ArtToday, Inc.

References

Abbeduto, L., & Hagerman, R. J. (1997). Language and communication in fragile X syndrome. *Mental Retardation and Developmental Disabilities Research Reviews, 3*(4), 313-322.

Abbeduto, L., Murphy, M. M., Cawthon, S. W., Richmond, E. K., Weissman, M. D., Karadottir, S., et al. (2003). Receptive language skills of adolescents and young adults with Down or fragile X syndrome. *American Journal of Mental Retardation, 108*(3), 149-160.

Abbeduto, L., Pavetto, M., Kesin, E., Weissman, M. D., Karadottir, S., O'Brien, A., et al. (2001). The linguistic and cognitive profile of Down syndrome: Evidence from a comparison with fragile X syndrome. *Down Syndrome Research and Practice, 7*(1), 9-15.

Achenbach, T. (1991). *Child behavior checklist for ages 4-18*. Burlington, VT: University of Vermont.

Allan, W., & Herndon, C. N. (1944). Retinitis pigmentosa and apparently sex-linked idiocy. *Journal of Heredity, 35*, 41-43.

Allan, W., Herndon, C. N., & Dudley, F. (1944). Some examples of the inheritance of mental deficiency: Apparently sex-linked idiocy and microcephaly. *American Journal of Mental Deficiency, 48*(4), 325-334.

Allingham-Hawkins, D. J., Babul-Hirji, R., Chitayat, D., Holden, J. J., Yang, K. T., Lee, C., et al. (1999). Fragile X premutation is a significant risk factor for premature ovarian failure: The International Collaborative POF in Fragile X study—Preliminary data. *American Journal of Medical Genetics, 83*(4), 322-325.

American Psychiatric Association (1994). *Diagnostic and statistical manual of mental disorders* (4th ed.). Washington DC: Author.

Anderson, W., Chitwood, S. & Hayden, D. (1997). *Negotiating the special education maze: A guide for parents and teachers*. Bethesda: Woodbine House.

Ayers, J. (1979). *Sensory integration and the child*. Los Angeles: Western Psychological Services.

Bailey, D. B., Jr., Hatton, D. D., Skinner, M., & Mesibov, G. (2001). Autistic behavior, FMR1 protein, and developmental trajectories in young males with fragile X syndrome. *Journal of Autism and Developmental Disorders, 31*(2), 165-174.

Bailey, D. B., Jr., Hatton, D. D., Tassone, F., Skinner, M., & Taylor, A. K. (2001). Variability in FMRP and early development in males with fragile X syndrome. *American Journal of Mental Retardation, 106*(1), 16-27.

Bailey, D. B., Jr., Roberts, J. E., Mirrett, P., & Hatton, D. D. (2001). Identifying infants and toddlers with fragile X syndrome: Issues and recommendations. *Infants and Young Children, 14*(1), 24-33.

Bailey, D. B., Jr., Skinner, D., & Sparkman, K. L. (2003). Discovering fragile X syndrome: Family experiences and perceptions. *Pediatrics, 111*(2), 407-416.

Bailey, D. B., Jr., Skinner, D., Sparkman, K. L., Moore, C. A., Olney, R. S., & Crawford, D. C. (2002). Delayed diagnosis of fragile X syndrome—United States, 1990-1999. *Morbidity and Mortality Weekly Report, 51*(33), 740-742.

Bakker, C. E., Kooy, R. F., D'Hooge, R., Tamanini, F., Willemsen, R., Nieuwenhuizen, I., et al. (2000). Introduction of a FMR1 transgene in the fragile X knockout mouse. *Neuroscience Research Communications, 26*(3), 265-277.

Baranek, G. T., Chin, Y. H., Hess, L. M., Yankee, J. G., Hatton, D. D., & Hooper, S. R. (2002). Sensory processing correlates of occupational performance in children with fragile X syndrome: Preliminary findings. *American Journal of Occupational Therapy, 56*(5), 538-546.

Barnett, B. G., Crews, C. J., & Douglas, J. T. (2002). Targeted adenoviral vectors. *Biochimica et Biophysica Acta, 1575*, 1-14.

Belser, R. C., & Sudhalter, V. (1995). Arousal difficulties in males with fragile X syndrome: A preliminary report. *Developmental Brain Dysfunction, 8*(4-6), 270-279.

Belser, R. C., & Sudhalter, V. (2001). Conversational characteristics of children with fragile X syndrome: Repetitive speech. *American Journal of Mental Retardation, 106*(1), 28-38.

Bennetto, L. & Pennington, B. (2002). Neuropsychology. In R. J. Hagerman & P. J. Hagerman (Eds.). *Fragile X syndrome: Diagnosis, treatment and research* (pp. 206-250). Baltimore: Johns Hopkins University Press.

Bennetto, L., Pennington, B. F., Porter, D., Taylor, A. K., & Hagerman, R. J. (2001). Profile of cognitive functioning in women with the fragile X mutation. *Neuropsychology, 15*(2), 290-299.

Berry-Kravis, E. (2002). Epilepsy in fragile X syndrome. *Developmental Medicine and Child Neurology, 44*(11), 724-728.

Berry-Kravis, E. (2003). Effects of ampakine CX516 on cognition and functioning in fragile X syndrome and autism. *FRAXA Update, 10*(2), 4.

Blackhurst, A. E., & Berdine, W. H. (1993). *An introduction to special education.* New York: Harper Collins.

Braden, M. (1989). *Logo reading system.* 100 E. St. Vrain, #200, Colorado Springs, CO.

Braden, M. (2000a). *Curriculum guide for Individuals with fragile X syndrome.* 100 E. St. Vrain, #200, Colorado Springs, CO.

Braden, M. (2000b). *Fragile: Handle with care, more about fragile X syndrome.* Colorado Springs: Spectra Publishing Co., Inc.

Braden, M. (2002a). Academic interventions. In R. J. Hagerman & P. J. Hagerman (Eds.). *Fragile X syndrome: Diagnosis, treatment and research* (3rd ed., pp. 287-338). Baltimore: Johns Hopkins University Press, 428-464.

Braden, M. (2002b). Helping cautious caterpillars turn into social butterflies: Social skills at home, at work, and at school. *Conference Proceedings: Eighth International Conference of the National Fragile X Foundation.* San Francisco: National Fragile X Foundation.

Braden, M. (2002c). The raging age: How to treat aggressive behaviors. *Conference Proceedings: Eighth International Conference of the National Fragile X Foundation.* San Francisco: National Fragile X Foundation.

Brainard, S. S., Schreiner, R. A., & Hagerman, R. J. (1991). Cognitive profiles of the carrier fragile X woman. *American Journal of Medical Genetics, 38*(2-3), 505-508.

Brown, W. T. (2002). The molecular biology of the fragile X mutation. In R. J. Hagerman & P. J. Hagerman (Eds.), *Fragile X syndrome: Diagnosis, treatment and research* (3rd ed., pp. 110-135). Baltimore: Johns Hopkins University Press.

Butler, M. G., Allen, A., Singh, D. N., Carpenter, N. J., & Hall, B. D. (1988). Photoanthropometric analysis of individuals with the fragile X syndrome. *American Journal of Medical Genetics, 30*(1-2), 165-168.

Butler, M. G., Brunschwig, A., Miller, L. K., & Hagerman, R. J. (1992). Standards for selected anthropometric measurements in males with the fragile X syndrome. *Pediatrics, 89*(6 Pt 1), 1059-1062.

Butler, M. G., Pratesi, R., Watson, M. S., Breg, W. R., & Singh, D. N. (1993). Anthropometric and craniofacial patterns in mentally retarded males with emphasis on the fragile X syndrome. *Clinical Genetics, 44*(3), 129-138.

Cantú, J. M., Scaglia, H. E., Medina, M., González-Diddi, M., Morato, T., Moreno, M. E., et al. (1976). Inherited congenital normofunctional testicular hyperplasia and mental deficiency. *Human Genetics, 33*(1), 23-33.

Carrow-Woolfolk, E. (1985). *Test for auditory comprehension of language-Revised.* Austin, TX: Pro-Ed.

Castrén, M., Pääkkönen, A., Tarkka, I. M., Ryynänen, M., & Partanen, J. (2003). Augmentation of auditory N1 in children with fragile X syndrome. *Brain Topography, 15*(3), 165-171.

Children's Health Act of 2000, H.R. 4365, 106th Cong. (2000).

Chiurazzi, P., Hamel, B. C. J., & Neri, G. (2001). XLMR genes: Update 2000. *European Journal of Human Genetics, 9*, 71-81.

Chiurazzi, P., Pomponi, M. G., Pietrobono, R., Bakker, C. E., Neri, G., & Oostra, B. A. (1999). Synergistic effect of histone hyperacetylation and DNA demethylation in the reactivation of the FMR1 gene. *Human Molecular Genetics, 8*(12), 2317-2323.

Churchill, J. D., Grossman, A. W., Irwin, S. A., Galvez, R., Klintsova, A. Y., Weiler, I. J., et al. (2002). A converging-methods approach to fragile X syndrome. *Developmental Psychobiology, 40*(3), 323-338.

Coffee, B., Zhang, F., Warren, S. T., & Reines, D. (1999). Acetylated histones are associated with FMR1 in normal but not fragile X-syndrome cells [published erratum appears in Nature Genetics 1999 Jun;22(2):209]. *Nature Genetics, 22*(1), 98-101.

Comery, T. A., Harris, J. B., Willems, P. J., Oostra, B. A., Irwin, S. A., Weiler, I. J., et al. (1997). Abnormal dendritic spines in fragile X knockout mice: maturation and pruning deficits. *Proceedings of the National Academy of Sciences of the United States of America, 94*(10), 5401-5404.

Cossée, M., Moutou, C., Biancalana, V., Bouix, J. C., Plessis, G., Delobel, B., et al. (1997). Le syndrome X fragile est encore méconnu: Efficacité du diagnostic moléculaire chez les proposants avec retard mental [Fragile X syndrome is still unrecognized: Efficacy of molecular diagnosis in mentally retarded probands]. *Archives de Pédiatrie, 4*(3), 227-236.

Crabbe, L. S., Bensky, A. S., Hornstein, L., & Schwartz, D. C. (1993). Cardiovascular abnormalities in children with fragile X syndrome. *Pediatrics, 91*(4), 714-715.

Davids, J. R., Hagerman, R. J., & Eilert, R. E. (1990). Orthopaedic aspects of fragile-X syndrome. *Journal of Bone and Joint Surgery, 72*(6), 889-896.

De Carli, L., Boncinelli, E., Danieli, G. A., & Larizza, L. (1998). *Genetica generale e umana* (Vol. II). Padova, Italy: Piccin.

de Vries, B. B., Fryns, J. P., Butler, M. G., Canziani, F., Wesby-van Swaay, E., van Hemel, J. O., et al. (1993). Clinical and molecular studies in fragile X patients with a Prader-Willi-like phenotype. *Journal of Medical Genetics, 30*(9), 761-766.

de Vries, B. B., Robinson, H., Stolte-Dijkstra, I., Tjon Pian Gi, C. V., Dijkstra, P. F., van Doorn, J., et al. (1995). General overgrowth in the fragile X syndrome: Variability in the phenotypic expression of the FMR1 gene mutation. *Journal of Medical Genetics, 32*(10), 764-769.

de Vries, B. B., Wiegers, A. M., Smits, A. P., Mohkamsing, S., Duivenvoorden, H. J., Fryns, J. P., et al. (1996). Mental status of females with an FMR1 gene full mutation. *American Journal of Human Genetics, 58*(5), 1025-1032.

Devys, D., Lutz, Y., Rouyer, N., Bellocq, J. P., & Mandel, J. L. (1993). The FMR-1 protein is cytoplasmic, most abundant in neurons and appears normal in carriers of a fragile X premutation. *Nature Genetics, 4*(4), 335-340.

Dyer-Friedman, J., Glaser, B., Hessl, D., Johnston, C., Huffman, L. C., Taylor, A., et al. (2002). Genetic and environmental influences on the cognitive outcomes of children with fragile X syndrome. *Journal of the American Academy of Child and Adolescent Psychiatry, 41*(3), 237-244.

Dykens, E. M., Hodapp, R. M., & Leckman, J. F. (1994). *Behavior and development in fragile X syndrome.* Thousand Oaks, CA: Sage Publications.

Feinstein, C., & Reiss, A. L. (1998). Autism: The point of view from fragile X studies. *Journal of Autism and Developmental Disorders, 28*(5), 393-405.

Fisch, G. S. (1993). What is associated with the fragile X syndrome? *American Journal of Medical Genetics, 48*(2), 112-121.

Fisch, G. S., Holden, J. J., Carpenter, N. J., Howard-Peebles, P. N., Maddalena, A., Pandya, A., et al. (1999). Age-related language characteristics of children and adolescents with fragile X syndrome. *American Journal of Medical Genetics, 83*(4), 253-256.

Fisch, G. S., Shapiro, L. R., Simensen, R., Schwartz, C. E., Fryns, J. P., Borghgraef, M., et al. (1992). Longitudinal changes in IQ among fragile X males: Clinical evidence of more than one mutation? *American Journal of Medical Genetics, 43*(1-2), 28-34.

Freund, L. S., Peebles, C. D., Aylward, E., & Reiss, A. L. (1995). Preliminary report on cognitive and adaptive behaviors of preschool-aged males with fragile X. *Developmental Brain Dysfunction, 8*(4-6), 242-251.

Freund, L. S., & Reiss, A. L. (1991). Cognitive profiles associated with the fra(X) syndrome in males and females. *American Journal of Medical Genetics, 38*(4), 542-547.

Fryns, J.P. (1985). X-linked mental retardation. In *Medical genetics: Past, present and future* (pp. 309-319). New York: Alan R. Liss.

Fryns, J. P., Moerman, P., Gilis, F., d'Espallier, L., & Van den Berghe, H. (1988). Suggestively increased rate of infant death in children of fra(X) positive mothers. *American Journal of Medical Genetics, 30*(1-2), 73-75.

Gagnon, E. (2001). Power cards: Using special interests to motivate children and youth with Asperger syndrome and autism. Shawnee Mission, KS: Autism Asperger Publishing Co.

Gane, L. W., & Cronister, A. (2002). Genetic Counseling. In R. J. Hagerman & P. J. Hagerman (Eds.), *Fragile X syndrome: Diagnosis, treatment, and research* (3rd ed., pp. 251-286). Baltimore: Johns Hopkins University Press.

Giraud, F., Ayme, S., Mattei, J. F., & Mattei, M. G. (1976). Constitutional chromosomal breakage. *Human Genetics, 34*(2), 125-136.

Goddard, H. H. (1914). *Feeble-mindedness. Its causes and consequences.* New York: MacMillan.

Gray, C. (1995). Teaching children with autism to "read" social situations. In K. Quill (ed.). *Teaching children with autism: Strategies to enhance communication and socialization* (pp. 219-241). Albany, NY: Delmar.

Greco, C. M., Hagerman, R. J., Tassone, F., Chudley, A. E., Del Bigio, M. R., Jacquemont, S., et al. (2002). Neuronal intranuclear inclusions in a new cerebellar tremor/ataxia syndrome among fragile X carriers. *Brain, 125*(Pt 8), 1760-1771.

Grilley, B. J., & Gee, A. P. (2003). Gene transfer: Regulatory issues and their impact on the clinical investigator and the good manufacturing production facility. *Cytotherapy, 5*(3), 197-207.

Hagerman, P. (2002). FMR1 gene expression and prospects for gene therapy. In R. J. Hagerman & P. J. Hagerman (Eds.), *Fragile X syndrome: Diagnosis, treatment, and research* (3rd ed., pp. 465-494). Baltimore: Johns Hopkins University Press.

Hagerman, R. (2002a). Medical follow-up and pharmacotherapy. In R. J. Hagerman & P. J. Hagerman (Eds.), *Fragile X syndrome: Diagnosis, treatment, and research* (3rd ed., pp. 287-338). Baltimore: Johns Hopkins University Press.

Hagerman, R. (2002b). The physical and behavioral phenotype. In R. J. Hagerman & P. J. Hagerman (Eds.), *Fragile X syndrome: Diagnosis, treatment, and research* (3rd ed., pp. 3-109). Baltimore: Johns Hopkins University Press.

Hagerman, R. J., Altshul-Stark, D., & McBogg, P. (1987). Recurrent otitis media in the fragile X syndrome. *American Journal of Diseases of Children, 141*(2), 184-187.

Hagerman, R. J., Hills, J., Scharfenaker, S., & Lewis, H. (1999). Fragile X syndrome and selective mutism. *American Journal of Medical Genetics, 83*(4), 313-317.

Hagerman, R. J., Leehey, M., Heinrichs, W., Tassone, F., Wilson, R., Hills, J., et al. (2001). Intention tremor, parkinsonism, and generalized brain atrophy in male carriers of fragile X. *Neurology, 57*(1), 127-130.

Hagerman, R. J., & Synhorst, D. P. (1984). Mitral valve prolapse and aortic dilatation in the fragile X syndrome. *American Journal of Medical Genetics, 17*(1), 123-131.

Hagerman, R. J., Van Housen, K., Smith, A. C., & McGavran, L. (1984). Consideration of connective tissue dysfunction in the fragile X syndrome. *American Journal of Medical Genetics, 17*(1), 111-121.

Harris-Schmidt, G., & Fast, D. (1998). Fragile X syndrome: Genetics, characteristics, and educational implications. *Advances in Special Education, 11*, 187-222.

Harvey, J., Judge, C., & Wiener, S. (1977). Familial X-linked mental retardation with an X chromosome abnormality. *Journal of Medical Genetics, 14*(1), 46-50.

Hatton, D. D., Hooper, S. R., Bailey, D. B., Skinner, M. L., Sullivan, K. M., & Wheeler, A. (2002). Problem behavior in boys with fragile X syndrome. *American Journal of Medical Genetics, 108*(2), 105-116.

Hay, D. A. (1994). Does IQ decline with age in fragile-X? A methodological critique. *American Journal of Medical Genetics, 51*(4), 358-363.

Heine-Suner, D., Torres-Juan, L., Morla, M., Busquets, X., Barcelo, F., Pico, G., et al. (2003). Fragile-X syndrome and skewed X-chromosome inactivation within a family: A female member with complete inactivation of the functional X chromosome. *American Journal of Medical Genetics, 122A*(2), 108-114.

Hessl, D., Dyer-Friedman, J., Glaser, B., Wisbeck, J., Barajas, R. G., Taylor, A., et al. (2001). The influence of environmental and genetic factors on behavior problems and autistic symptoms in boys and girls with fragile X syndrome. *Pediatrics, 108*(5), 1-9.

Hills Epstein, J., Riley, K., & Sobesky, W. (2002). The treatment of emotional and behavioral problems. In R. J. Hagerman & P. J. Hagerman (Eds.), *Fragile X syndrome: Diagnosis, treatment and research* (3rd ed., pp. 339-362). Baltimore: Johns Hopkins University Press.

Hockey, A., & Crowhurst, J. (1988). Early manifestations of the Martin-Bell syndrome based on a series of both sexes from infancy. *American Journal of Medical Genetics, 30*(1-2), 61-71.

Hodapp, R. M., DesJardin, J. L., & Ricci, L. A. (2003). Genetic syndromes of mental retardation. Should they matter for the early interventionist? *Infants and Young Children, 16*(2), 152-160.

Holliday, R. (1993). Epigenetic inheritance based on DNA methylation. In J. P. Jost & H. P. Saluz (Eds.), *DNA methylation: Molecular biology and biological significance* (Vol. 64, pp. 452-468). Basel, Switzerland: Birkhäuser Verlag.

Hull, C., & Hagerman, R. J. (1993). A study of the physical, behavioral, and medical phenotype, including anthropometric measures, of females with fragile X syndrome. *American Journal of Diseases of Children, 147*(11), 1236-1241.

Hundscheid, R. D., Smits, A. P., Thomas, C. M., Kiemeney, L. A., & Braat, D. D. (2003). Female carriers of fragile X premutations have no increased risk for additional diseases other than premature ovarian failure. *American Journal of Medical Genetics, 117A*(1), 6-9.

Irwin, S. A., Patel, B., Idupulapati, M., Harris, J. B., Crisostomo, R. A., Larsen, B. P., et al. (2001). Abnormal dendritic spine characteristics in the temporal and visual cortices of patients with fragile-X syndrome: a quantitative examination. *American Journal of Medical Genetics, 98*(2), 161-167.

Jacquemont, S., Hagerman, R. J., Leehey, M., Grigsby, J., Zhang, L., Brunberg, J. A., et al. (2003). Fragile X premutation tremor/ataxia syndrome: Molecular, clinical, and neuroimaging correlates. *American Journal of Human Genetics, 72*(4), 869-878.

Johnson, D. & Myklebust, H. (1967). *Learning disabilities: Educational principles and practices.* New York: Grune and Stratton.

Johnson, G. E. (1897). Contribution to the psychology and pedagogy of feeble-minded children. *Journal of Psycho-asthenics, 2,* 26-32.

Johnson-Glenberg, M.C. (2003). *Reading skill and working memory in those with fragile X syndrome.* Paper presented at the 25th Annual Symposium on Research in Child Language Disorders, Madison, WI.

Kaufman, A. & Kaufman, N. (1983). *Kaufman-Assessment Battery for Children.* Circle Pines, MN: American Guidance Service.

Kemper, M. B., Hagerman, R. J., & Altshul-Stark, D. (1988). Cognitive profiles of boys with the fragile X syndrome. *American Journal of Medical Genetics, 30*(1-2), 191-200.

Kenneson, A., Zhang, F., Hagedorn, C. H., & Warren, S. T. (2001). Reduced FMRP and increased FMR1 transcription is proportionally associated with CGG repeat number in intermediate-length and premutation carriers. *Human Molecular Genetics, 10*(14), 1449-1454.

Keysor, C. S., Mazzocco, M. M., McLeod, D. R., & Hoehn-Saric, R. (2002). Physiological arousal in females with fragile X or Turner syndrome. *Developmental Psychobiology, 41*(2), 133-146.

Kjaer, I., Hjalgrim, H., & Russell, B. G. (2001). Cranial and hand skeleton in fragile X syndrome. *American Journal of Medical Genetics, 100*(2), 156-161.

Kluger, G., Bohm, I., Laub, M. C., & Waldenmaier, C. (1996). Epilepsy and fragile X gene mutations. *Pediatric Neurology, 15*(4), 358-360.

Kotilainen, J., & Pirinen, S. (1999). Dental maturity is advanced in fragile X syndrome. *American Journal of Medical Genetics, 83*(4), 298-301.

Kowalczyk, C. L., Schroeder, E., Pratt, V., Conard, J., Wright, K., & Feldman, G. L. (1996). An association between precocious puberty and fragile X syndrome? *Journal of Pediatric and Adolescent Gynecology, 9*(4), 199-202.

Kwon, H., Menon, V., Eliez, S., Warsofsky, I. S., White, C. D., Dyer-Friedman, J., et al. (2001). Functional neuroanatomy of visuospatial working memory in fragile X syndrome: Relation to behavioral and molecular measures. *American Journal of Psychiatry, 158*(7), 1040-1051.

Lachiewicz, A. M., & Dawson, D. V. (1994). Do young boys with fragile X syndrome have macroorchidism? *Pediatrics, 93*(6 Pt 1), 992-995.

Laggerbauer, B., Ostareck, D., Keidel, E.-M., Ostareck-Lederer, A., & Fischer, U. (2001). Evidence that fragile X mental retardation protein is a negative regulator of translation. *Human Molecular Genetics, 10*(4), 329-338.

Laird, C. D. (1991). Possible erasure of the imprint on a fragile X chromosome when transmitted by a male. *American Journal of Medical Genetics, 38*(2-3), 391-395.

Lauterborn, J. C. (2003). Effects of positive AMPA receptor modulation in the FMR1 knockout mouse. *FRAXA Update, 10*(2), 4.

Lauterborn, J. C., Truong, G. S., Baudry, M., Bi, X., Lynch, G., & Gall, C. M. (2003). Chronic elevation of brain-derived neurotrophic factor by ampakines. *Journal of Pharmacology and Experimental Therapeutics, 307*(1), 297-305.

Leifert, J. A., & Whitton, J. L. (2003). "Translocatory proteins" and "protein transduction domains": A critical analysis of their biological effects and the underlying mechanisms. *Molecular Therapy, 8*(1), 13-20.

Lipps, H. J., Jenke, A. C. W., Nehlsen, K., Scinteie, M. F., Stehle, I. M., & Bode, J. (2003). Chromosome-based vectors for gene therapy. *Gene, 304*, 23-33.

Lisik, M., Szymanska-Parkieta, K., & Galecka, U. (2000). The comparison of anthropometric variables in mentally retarded boys with and without fragile X syndrome. *Clinical Genetics, 57*(6), 456-458.

Loesch, D. Z., & Hay, D. A. (1988). Clinical features and reproductive patterns in fragile X female heterozygotes. *Journal of Medical Genetics, 25*(6), 407-414.

Loesch, D. Z., Lafranchi, M., & Scott, D. (1988). Anthropometry in Martin-Bell syndrome. *American Journal of Medical Genetics, 30*(1-2), 149-164.

Loesch, D. Z., & Sampson, M. L. (1993). Effect of the fragile X anomaly on body proportions estimated by pedigree analysis. *Clinical Genetics, 44*(2), 82-88.

Lubs, H. A. (1969). A marker X chromosome. *American Journal of Human Genetics, 21*, 231-244.

Lucock, M. (2000). Folic acid: Nutritional biochemistry, molecular biology, and role in disease processes. *Molecular Genetics and Metabolism, 71*, 121-138.

Lundberg, M., Wikström, S., & Johansson, M. (2003). Cell surface adherence and endocytyosis of protein transduction domains. *Molecular Therapy, 8*(1), 143-150.

Lyon, M. F. (1962). Sex chromatin and gene action in the mammalian X-chromosome. *American Journal of Human Genetics, 14*, 135-148.

Maes, B., Fryns, J. P., Van Walleghem, M., & Van den Berghe, H. (1994). Cognitive functioning and information processing of adult mentally retarded men with fragile-X syndrome. *American Journal of Medical Genetics, 50*(2), 190-200.

Martin, J. P., & Bell, J. (1943). A pedigree of mental defect showing sex-linkage. *Journal of Neurology and Psychiatry, 6*, 154-167.

Mazzocco, M. M. (2001). Math learning disability and math LD subtypes: Evidence from studies of Turner syndrome, fragile X syndrome, and neurofibromatosis type 1. *Journal of Learning Disabilities, 34*(6), 520-533.

Mazzocco, M. M., Hagerman, R. J., & Pennington, B. F. (1992). Problem solving limitations among cytogenetically expressing fragile X women. *American Journal of Medical Genetics, 43*(1-2), 78-86.

Mazzocco, M. & Lachiewicz, A. (2003). Education strategies in math. *Conference Proceedings: Eighth International Conference of the National Fragile X Foundation*. San Francisco: National Fragile X Foundation.

McCarthy, (1972). *McCarthy Scales of Children's Ability*. San Antonio: The Psychological Corporation.

Mirrett, P, Roberts, J., & Price, J. (2003). Early intervention practices and communication intervention strategies for young males with fragile X syndrome. *Language, Speech and Hearing Services in Schools, 34*(4), 320-331.

Moore-Brown, B. & Montgomery, J. (2001). *Making a difference for America's children: Speech-language pathologists in the public schools*. Eau Claire: Thinking Publications.

Morgan, T. H. (1910). Sex limited inheritance in Drosophila. *Science, 32*, 120-122.

Murphy, M. M., & Abbeduto, L. (2003). Language and communication in fragile X syndrome. In L. Abbeduto (Ed.), *International Review of Research in Mental Retardation: Vol. 27. Language and communication in mental retardation* (pp. 83-119). New York: Academic Press.

Murray, A., Ennis, S., MacSwiney, F., Webb, J., & Morton, N. E. (2000). Reproductive and menstrual history of females with fragile X expansions. *European Journal of Human Genetics, 8*(4), 247-252.

Musumeci, S. A., Ferri, R., Elia, M., Dal Gracco, S., Scuderi, C., Stefanini, M., et al. (1995). Sleep neurophysiology in fragile X patients. *Developmental Brain Dysfunction, 8*(4-6), 218-222.

Myers, G. F., Mazzoco, M. M., Maddalena, A., & Reiss, A. L. (2001). No widespread psychological effect of the fragile X premutation in childhood: Evidence from a preliminary controlled study. *Journal of Developmental and Behavioral Pediatrics, 22*(6), 353-359.

Nimchinsky, E. A., Oberlander, A. M., & Svoboda, K. (2001). Abnormal development of dendritic spines in FMR1 knock-out mice. *Journal of Neuroscience, 21*(14), 5139-5146.

Nolin, S. L., Brown, W. T., Glicksman, A., Houck, G. E., Jr., Gargano, A. D., Sullivan, A., et al. (2003). Expansion of the fragile X CGG repeat in females with premutation or intermediate alleles. *American Journal of Human Genetics, 72*(2), 454-464.

Nolin, S. L., Lewis, F. A., 3rd, Ye, L. L., Houck, G. E., Jr., Glicksman, A. E., Limprasert, P., et al. (1996). Familial transmission of the FMR1 CGG repeat. *American Journal of Human Genetics, 59*(6), 1252-1261.

Office of Biotechnology Activities. (2003). *Human gene transfer protocols*. Bethesda, MD: National Institutes of Health.

Ohashi, S., Kubo, T., Kishida, T., Ikeda, T., Takahashi, K., Arai, Y., et al. (2002). Successful genetic transduction in vivo into synovium by means of electroporation. *Biochemical and Biophysical Research Communications, 293*, 1530-1535.

Opitz, J. M., Westphal, J. M., & Daniel, A. (1984). Discovery of a connective tissue dysplasia in the Martin-Bell syndrome. *American Journal of Medical Genetics, 17*(1), 101-109.

Partington, M. W. (1984). The fragile X syndrome II: Preliminary data on growth and development in males. *American Journal of Medical Genetics, 17*(1), 175-194.

Partington, M. W., Robinson, H., Laing, S., & Turner, G. (1992). Mortality in the fragile X syndrome: Preliminary data. *American Journal of Medical Genetics, 43*(1-2), 120-123.

Pearson, C. E., Eichler, E. E., Lorenzetti, D., Kramer, S. F., Zoghbi, H. Y., Nelson, D. L., et al. (1998). Interruptions in the triplet repeats of SCA1 and FRAXA reduce the propensity and complexity of slipped strand DNA (S-DNA) formation. *Biochemistry, 37*(8), 2701-2708.

Peier, A. M., McIlwain, K. L., Kenneson, A., Warren, S. T., Paylor, R., & Nelson, D. L. (2000). (Over)correction of FMR1 deficiency with YAC transgenics: Behavioral and physical features. *Human Molecular Genetics, 9*(8), 1145-1159.

Peretz, B., Ever-Hadani, P., Casamassimo, P., Eidelman, E., Shellhart, C., & Hagerman, R. (1988). Crown size asymmetry in males with fra (X) or Martin-Bell syndrome. *American Journal of Medical Genetics, 30*(1-2), 185-190.

Pierangelo, R. & Crane, R. (1997). *Complete guide to special education transition services*. West Nyack: The Center for Applied Research in Education.

Richard, G. (2001). *The source for processing disorders*. East Moline, IL: LinguiSystems.

Richards, B. W., Sylvester, P. E., & Brooker, C. (1981). Fragile X-linked mental retardation: The Martin-Bell syndrome. *Journal of Mental Deficiency Research, 25 Pt 4*, 253-256.

Riddle, J. E., Cheema, A., Sobesky, W. E., Gardner, S. C., Taylor, A. K., Pennington, B. F., et al. (1998). Phenotypic involvement in females with the FMR1 gene mutation. *American Journal on Mental Retardation, 102*(6), 590-601.

Rivera, S. M., Menon, V., White, C. D., Glaser, B., & Reiss, A. L. (2002). Functional brain activation during arithmetic processing in females with fragile X syndrome is related to FMR1 protein expression. *Human Brain Mapping, 16*(4), 206-218.

Roberts, J. E., Boccia, M. L., Bailey, D. B., Jr., Hatton, D. D., & Skinner, M. (2001). Cardiovascular indices of physiological arousal in boys with fragile X syndrome. *Developmental Psychobiology, 39*(2), 107-123.

Roberts, J. E., Mirrett, P., Anderson, K., Burchinal, M., & Neebe, E. (2002). Early communication, symbolic behavior, and social profiles of young males with fragile X syndrome. *American Journal of Speech-Language Pathology, 11*(3), 295-304.

Roberts, J. E., Mirrett, P., & Burchinal, M. (2001). Receptive and expressive communication development of young males with fragile X syndrome. *American Journal on Mental Retardation, 106*(3), 216-230.

Rogers, S. J., Wehner, E. A., & Hagerman, R. (2001). The behavioral phenotype in fragile X: Symptoms of autism in very young children with fragile X syndrome, idiopathic autism, and other developmental disorders. *Journal of Developmental & Behavioral Pediatrics, 22*(6), 409-417.

Rondal, J. & Edwards, S. (1997). *Language in mental retardation*. London: Whurr Publishers Ltd.

Rubanyi, G. M. (2001). The future of human gene therapy. *Molecular Aspects of Medicine, 22*(3), 113-142.

Ruvalcaba, R. H. A., Myhre, S. A., Roosen-Runge, E. C., & Beckwith, J. B. (1977). X-linked mental deficiency megalotestes syndrome. *JAMA, 238*(15), 1646-1650.

References

Sabaratnam, M., Vroegop, P. G., & Gangadharan, S. K. (2001). Epilepsy and EEG findings in 18 males with fragile X syndrome. *Seizure, 10*(1), 60-63.

Santos, K. E. (1992). Fragile X syndrome: An educator's role in identification, prevention, and intervention. *Remedial and Special Education, 13*(2), 32-39.

Saunders, S. (1999). Teaching children with fragile X syndrome. *British Journal of Special Education, 26*(2), 76-79.

Saunders, S. (2001). *Fragile X syndrome: A guide for teachers.* London: David Fulton Publishers.

Scharfenaker, S., O'Conner, R., Stackhouse, T., Braden, M. and Gray, K. (2002). An integrated approach to intervention. In R. J. Hagerman & P. J. Hagerman (Eds.). *Fragile X syndrome: Diagnosis, treatment and research* (3rd ed., pp. 363-427). Baltimore: Johns Hopkins University Press.

Schepis, C., Palazzo, R., Cannavo, S. P., Ragusa, R. M., Barletta, C., & Spina, E. (1990). Prevalence of primary cutis verticis gyrata in a psychiatric population: Association with chromosomal fragile sites. *ACTA Dermato-Venereologica (Oslo), 70*(6), 483-486.

Schoenbrodt, L. & Smith, R. (1995). Children with fragile X syndrome. In L. Schoenbrodt and R. Smith (Eds.). *Communication disorders and interventions in low incidence pediatric populations* (pp. 59-91). San Diego: Singular Publishing Group.

Schultz-Pedersen, S., Hasle, H., Olsen, J. H., & Friedrich, U. (2001). Evidence of decreased risk of cancer in individuals with fragile X. *American Journal of Medical Genetics, 103*(3), 226-230.

Senner, J. (2002). Introduction to AAC. *Proceedings of the Eighth International Fragile X Conference.* San Francisco: National Fragile X Foundation.

Sherman, S. L. (2002). Epidemiology. In R. J. Hagerman & P. J. Hagerman (Eds.), *Fragile X syndrome: Diagnosis, treatment, and research* (3rd ed., pp. 136-168). Baltimore: Johns Hopkins University Press.

Simko, A., Hornstein, L., Soukup, S., & Bagamery, N. (1989). Fragile X syndrome: Recognition in young children. *Pediatrics, 83*(4), 547-552.

Slegtenhorst-Eegdeman, K. E., de Rooij, D. G., Verhoef-Post, M., van de Kant, H. J., Bakker, C. E., Oostra, B. A., et al. (1998). Macroorchidism in FMR1 knockout mice is caused by increased Sertoli cell proliferation during testicular development. *Endocrinology, 139*(1), 156-162.

Smith, S.E. (1993). Cognitive deficits associated with fragile X syndrome. *Mental Retardation, 31*(5), 279-283.

Snow, J. & Hasbury, D. (1989). The circle of friends. In *Action for inclusion: How to improve schools by welcoming children with special needs into regular classrooms.* Toronto: Inclusion Press.

Sobesky, W. E., Pennington, B. F., Porter, D., Hull, C. E., & Hagerman, R. J. (1994). Emotional and neurocognitive deficits in fragile X. *American Journal of Medical Genetics, 51*(4), 378-385.

Sobesky, W. E., Porter, D., Pennington, B. F., & Hagerman, R. J. (1995). Dimensions of shyness in fragile X females. *Developmental Brain Dysfunction, 8*(4-6), 340-345.

Spiridigliozzi, G. A., Lachiewicz, A., MacMurdo, C., Vizoso, A., O'Donnell, C., Conkie-Russell, A., et al. (1994). *Educating boys with fragile X syndrome : A guide for parents and professionals.* Durham N.C.: Duke University Medical Center Child Development Unit.

Stackhouse, T. and Scharfenacker, S. (2002). Combining occupational therapy and speech. *Proceedings of the Eighth International Fragile X Conference.* San Francisco: National Fragile X Foundation.

Steiger, C. (1998). *My brother has fragile X*. Chapel Hill: Avanta Media Corporation.

Stolberg, S. G. (1999, 28 November 1999). The biotech death of Jesse Gelsinger. *New York Times Magazine*, p. 137.

Stoll, C. (2001). Problems in the diagnosis of fragile X syndrome in young children are still present. *American Journal of Medical Genetics, 100*(2), 110-115.

Storm, R. L., PeBenito, R., & Ferretti, C. (1987). Ophthalmologic findings in the fragile X syndrome. *Archives of Ophthalmology, 105*(8), 1099-1102.

Sudhalter, V. (2002). Hyperarousal and inhibition problems in the speech and language of individuals with fragile X syndrome. *Proceedings of the Eighth International Fragile X Conference*. San Francisco: National Fragile X Foundation.

Sutherland, G. R. (1977). Fragile sites on human chromosomes: Demonstration of their dependence on the type of tissue culture medium. *Science, 197*(4300), 265-266.

Sutherland, G. R. (1979). Heritable fragile sites on human chromosomes I. Factors affecting expression in lymphocyte culture. *American Journal of Human Genetics, 31*(2), 125-135.

Symons, F. J., Clark, R. D., Hatton, D. D., Skinner, M., & Bailey, D. B., Jr. (2003). Self-injurious behavior in young boys with fragile X syndrome. *American Journal of Medical Genetics, 118A*(2), 115-121.

Symons, F. J., Clark, R. D., & Roberts, J. P. (2001). Classroom behavior of elementary school-age boys with fragile X syndrome. *The Journal of Special Education, 34*(4), 194-202.

Szymanski, C. (2003). *Developing opportunities to teach social skills*. Workshop presented for the South Cook County Cooperative for Special Education. Chicago, IL.

Tamm, L., Menon, V., Johnston, C. K., Hessl, D. R., & Reiss, A. L. (2002). FMRI study of cognitive interference processing in females with fragile X syndrome. *Journal of Cognitive Neuroscience, 14*(2), 160-171.

Tarleton, J. (2003). Detection of FMR1 trinucleotide repeat expansion mutations using Southern blot and PCR methodologies. In N. T. Potter (Ed.), *Methods in molecular biology: Vol. 217. Neurogenetics: Methods and protocols* (pp. 29-39). Totowa, NJ: Humana Press Inc.

Tassone, F., Hagerman, R. J., Chamberlain, W. D., & Hagerman, P. J. (2000). Transcription of the FMR1 gene in individuals with fragile X syndrome. *American Journal of Medical Genetics, 97*(3), 195-203.

Tassone, F., Hagerman, R. J., Taylor, A. K., Gane, L. W., Godfrey, T. E., & Hagerman, P. J. (2000). Elevated levels of FMR1 mRNA in carrier males: A new mechanism of involvement in the fragile-X syndrome. *American Journal of Human Genetics, 66*(1), 6-15.

Tassone, F., Hagerman, R. J., Taylor, A. K., & Hagerman, P. J. (2001). A majority of fragile X males with methylated, full mutation alleles have significant levels of FMR1 messenger RNA. *Journal of Medical Genetics, 38*(7), 453-456.

Thorndike, R., Hagen, E., & Sattler, J. (1985). *Stanford-Binet Intelligence Scale: Fourth edition*. Chicago: Riverside Publishing.

Turner, G., Eastman, C., Casey, J., McLeay, A., Procopis, P., & Turner, B. (1975). X-linked mental retardation associated with macro-orchidism. *Journal of Medical Genetics, 12*, 367-371.

Verkerk, A. J., Pieretti, M., Sutcliffe, J. S., Fu, Y. H., Kuhl, D. P., Pizzuti, A., et al. (1991). Identification of a gene (FMR-1) containing a CGG repeat coincident with a breakpoint cluster region exhibiting length variation in fragile X syndrome. *Cell, 65*(5), 905-914.

Vianna-Morgante, A. M. (1999). Twinning and premature ovarian failure in premutation fragile X carriers [letter]. *American Journal of Medical Genetics, 83*(4), 326.

Vygotsky, L.S. (1962). *Thought and language.* Cambridge: The MIT Press.

Waldstein, G., Mierau, G., Ahmad, R., Thibodeau, S. N., Hagerman, R. J., & Caldwell, S. (1987). Fragile X syndrome: Skin elastin abnormalities. *Birth Defects Original Article Series, 23*(1), 103-114.

Wechsler, D. (1974). *Wechsler Intelligence Scale for Children-Revised.* San Antonio: The Psychological Corporation.

Wechsler, D. (1981). *Wechsler Adult Intelligence Scale-Revised.* San Antonio: The Psychological Corporation.

Wilding, J., Cornish, K., & Munir, F. (2002). Further delineation of the executive deficit in males with fragile-X syndrome. *Neuropsychologia, 40*(8), 1343-1349.

Willemsen, R., Anar, B., Otero, Y. D., de Vries, B. B., Hilhorst-Hofstee, Y., Smits, A., et al. (1999). Noninvasive test for fragile X syndrome, using hair root analysis. *American Journal of Human Genetics, 65*(1), 98-103.

Williams, M. & Shellenberger, S. (1996). *How does your engine run? Alert program for self-regulation.* Albuquerque: Therapy Works.

Wren, C. (1983). Language and language disabilities. In C. Wren (Ed.) *Language learning disabilities: Diagnosis and remediation* (pp. 1-38). Rockville, MD: Aspen Publications.

Wren, C. (1985). Collecting language samples from children with syntax problems. *Language, Speech, and Hearing Services in Schools, 16,* 83-102.

Wright-Talamante, C., Cheema, A., Riddle, J. E., Luckey, D. W., Taylor, A. K., & Hagerman, R. J. (1996). A controlled study of longitudinal IQ changes in females and males with fragile X syndrome. *American Journal of Medical Genetics, 64*(2), 350-355.

Yorkston, K., Beukelman, D., Strand, E. & Bell, K. (1999). *Management of motor speech disorders in children and adults,* (2nd ed.). Austin: Pro-Ed.

Zhang, L., Nolan, E., Kreitschitz, S., & Rabussay, D. P. (2002). Enhanced delivery of naked DNA to the skin by non-invasive invivo electroporation. *Biochimica et Biophysica Acta, 1572,* 1-9.

Zhang, Y., Schlachetzki, F., & Pardridge, W. M. (2003). Global non-viral gene transfer to the primate brain following intravenous administration. *Molecular Therapy, 7*(1), 11-18.

Zhong, N., Yang, W., Dobkin, C., & Brown, W. T. (1995). Fragile X gene instability: Anchoring AGGs and linked microsatellites. *American Journal of Human Genetics, 57*(2), 351-361.

Websites

Apraxia Kids	http://www.apraxia-kids.org/
Carolina Fragile X Project	http://www.fpg.unc.edu/~fx/
FRAXA Research Foundation	http://www.fraxa.org/
National Fragile X Foundation	http://www.fragilex.org/

23-07-98765432